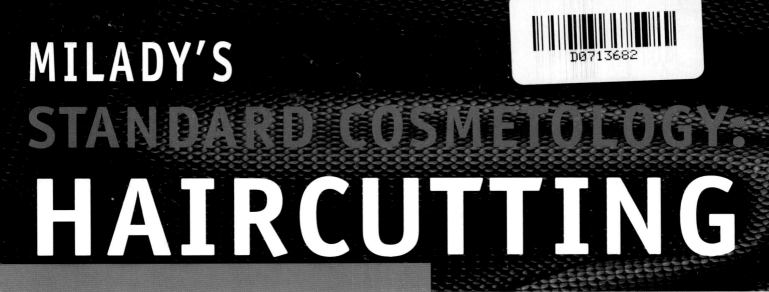

MILADY'S
STANDARD COSMETOLOGY:
HAIRCUTTING

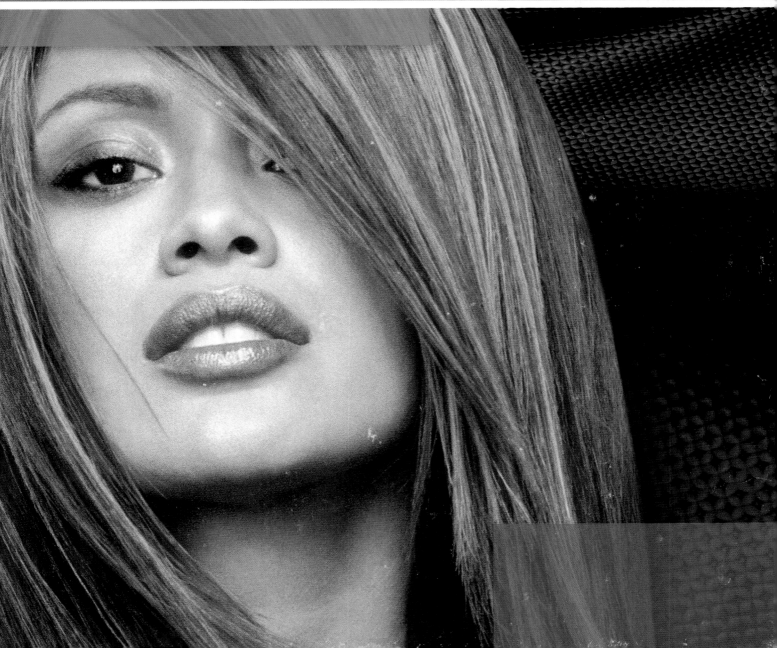

MILADY'S
STANDARD COSMETOLOGY:
HAIRCUTTING

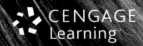

CENGAGE
Learning

Australia   Canada   Mexico   Singapore   Spain   United Kingdom   United States

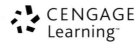

Milady's Standard Cosmetology: Haircutting
Compiled by Lisha Barnes

Vice President, Milady: Dawn Gerrain

Publisher: Erin O'Connor

Acquisitions Editor: Martine Edwards

Product Manager: Jessica Burns

Editorial Assistant: Mike Spring

Director of Beauty Industry Relations:
Sandra Bruce

Marketing Manager: Gerard McAvey

Production Director: Wendy Troeger

Senior Content Project Manager:
Nina Tucciarelli

Art Director: Joy Kocsis

Technology Project Manager: Sandy Charette

For product information and technology assistance, contact us at
Professional & Career Group Customer Support, 1-800-648-7450

For permission to use material from this text or product,
submit all requests online at **cengage.com/permissions**.
Further permissions questions can be e-mailed to
permissionrequest@cengage.com.

Library of Congress Control Number: 2006033202

ISBN-13: 978-1-4354-0074-0

ISBN-10: 1-4354-0074-7

Milady
5 Maxwell Drive
Clifton Park, NY 12065-2919
USA

Cengage Learning products are represented in Canada by Nelson Education, Ltd.

For your lifelong learning solutions, visit **delmar.cengage.com**
Visit our corporate website at **cengage.com**.

Notice to the Reader
Publisher does not warrant or guarantee any of the products described herein or perform any independent analysis in connection with any of the product information contained herein. Publisher does not assume, and expressly disclaims, any obligation to obtain and include information other than that provided to it by the manufacturer. The reader is expressly warned to consider and adopt all safety precautions that might be indicated by the activities described herein and to avoid all potential hazards. By following the instructions contained herein, the reader willingly assumes all risks in connection with such instructions. The publisher makes no representations or warranties of any kind, including but not limited to, the warranties of fitness for particular purpose or merchantability, nor are any such representations implied with respect to the material set forth herein, and the publisher takes no responsibility with respect to such material. The publisher shall not be liable for any special, consequential, or exemplary damages resulting, in whole or part, from the readers' use of, or reliance upon, this material.

Printed in Canada
3 4 5 XX 12 11 10 09

TABLE OF CONTENTS

v

PREFACE

Milady's Standard Cosmetology: Haircutting is a new, full-color, spiral-bound supplement to the leading cosmetology textbook *Milady's Standard Cosmetology*. This book provides you with step-by-step technicals for women's haircutting and hairstyling and for men's haircutting. Each technical features two categories: an overview and an apply. The overview is a short introduction providing a framework about the technique you will learn. The apply is the step-by-step part of the technique. Each step is explained in detail and is accompanied throughout by photos. Each technique will end with photos of the same technique performed on different hair lengths, colors, and textures to help ignite your imagination. This will help you consider different possibilities to applying what you've learned in many creative ways.

HAIRSTYLE IMAGE CREDITS

Create, pg. 9: Courtesy of Tom Carson, Bob Steele Salon, Atlanta, GA

Create, pg. 15: Courtesy of Tom Carson, Attitudes Salon, Toledo, OH

Create, pg. 21: Courtesy of Tom Carson, Savvy Salon, Cornelius, NC

Create, pg. 37: Courtesy of Tom Carson, Savvy Salon, Cornelius, NC

Create, pg. 37: Courtesy of Tom Carson, The Brown Aveda Institute, Mentor, OH

Create, pg. 37: Courtesy of Tom Carson, The Brown Aveda Institute, Mentor, OH

Blow-drying Horizontal Graduation, pg. 42: Courtesy of Tom Carson, Hair Benders Int'l, Chattanooga, TN

Create, pg. 45: Courtesy of Tom Carson, Bella Donna Salon, Painesville, OH

Create, pg. 45: Courtesy of Tom Carson, Above & Beyond Salon, Vermilion, OH

Blow-drying Layered Square Shape, pg. 50: Courtesy of Tom Carson, Sheer Professionals Salon, Wooster, OH

Create, pg. 52: Courtesy of Tom Carson, The Brown Aveda Institute, Mentor, OH

Create, pg. 52: Courtesy of Tom Carson, Ladies & Gentlemen Salon & Spa, Mentor, OH

Create, pg. 52: Courtesy of Tom Carson, Heavenly Hair, Indianapolis, IN

Create, pg. 52: Courtesy of Tom Carson, Shortino's, York, PA

Create, pg. 55: Courtesy of Tom Carson, Salon 2000, Indianapolis, IN

Create, pg. 55: Courtesy of Tom Carson, Shortino's, York, PA

Create, pg. 55: Courtesy of Tom Carson, Attitudes Salon, Toledo, OH

Create, pg. 59: Courtesy of Tom Carson, Yellow Strawberry Global Salons, Sarasota, FL

Create, pg. 59: Courtesy of Tom Carson, Shortino's, York, PA

Create, pg. 59: Courtesy of Tom Carson, Tangles Salon, Wichita Falls, TX

Create, pg. 65: Courtesy of Tom Carson, Above & Beyond Salon, Vermilion, OH

Create, pg. 65: Courtesy of Tom Carson, Jenniffer & Co. Salon, Mentor, OH

Press and Curl on Heavy Layers, pg. 69: Courtesy of Tom Carson, Sheer Professionals Salon, Wooster, OH

Create, pg. 73: Courtesy of Tom Carson, Sheer Professionals Salon, Wooster, OH

Wrapping Layered Graduation, pg. 83: Courtesy of Tom Carson, photo courtesy Salon Exclusive, Charlotte, NC. Hair by Maurice Lemmons. Make-up by Betty Mekonnen.

Create, pg. 85: Courtesy of Tom Carson, photo courtesy Salon Exclusive, Charlotte, NC. Hair by Maurice Lemmons. Make-up by Betty Mekonnen.

Create, pg. 91: Courtesy of Tom Carson, Kathy Adams Salon, Buford, GA

Create, pg. 91: Courtesy of Tom Carson, Kathy Adams Salon, Buford, GA

Create, pg. 91: Courtesy of Tom Carson, Jenniffer & Co. Salon, Mentor, OH

Create, pg. 91: Courtesy of Tom Carson, Kenneth's Hair With Style, Metairie, LA

Create, pg. 97: Courtesy of Tom Carson, Jenniffer & Co. Salon, Mentor, OH

Create, pg. 97: Courtesy of Tom Carson, Europa Salon, Beachwood, OH

Create, pg. 102: Courtesy of Tom Carson, Jenniffer & Co. Salon, Mentor, OH

Create, pg. 102: Courtesy of Tom Carson, Jenniffer & Co. Salon, Mentor, OH

WOMEN'S HAIRCUTTING

PART 1

HORIZONTAL BLUNT CUT

OVERVIEW

This is a smooth, sleek, and shiny shape that, when straight, contours to the curve of the head and has minimal volume, yet offers freedom of movement. When texture is added, the silhouette takes on a completely different look—it has enhanced volume and an expanded shape; the surface of the shape is of sculpted wave formations that create visual interest and a different type of energy. The result is a style quite different from sleek, smooth hair.

In this design, all hair lengths come to one hanging level, and the perimeter is horizontal.

APPLY

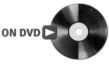
ON DVD ▶

With your clients, these technical steps will follow the consultation and shampoo.

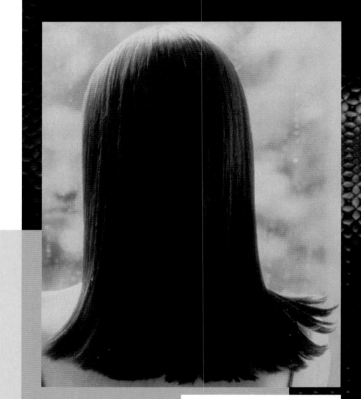

Shown above is the sleek, all one length horizontal blunt cut. Whether styled for symmetry or asymmetry, all lengths fall to one line.

PROCEDURE

1. Gently comb the wet hair. Create a natural part or an artificial part. To find the natural part, comb the hair back from the hairline at the forehead.

2. Push the hair forward until the natural part breaks. Comb the hair down from around natural part.

3. To create an artificial part, position the thumb at the natural crown area and the tip of the comb at the front hairline, then trace through from the front hairline to the crown.

4. Separate the hair so that the part is clearly visible.

5. Now move to the back and comb the hair into natural fall. Comb all around the crown, making certain all the hair is evenly distributed.

6. Part the back from the crown straight down to the nape, dividing the back into two equal sections.

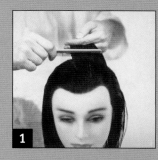

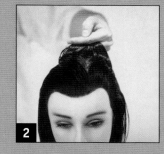

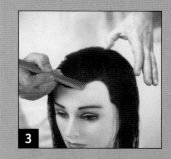

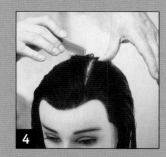

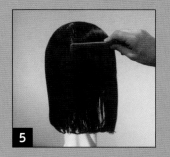

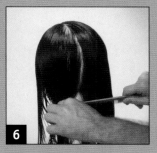

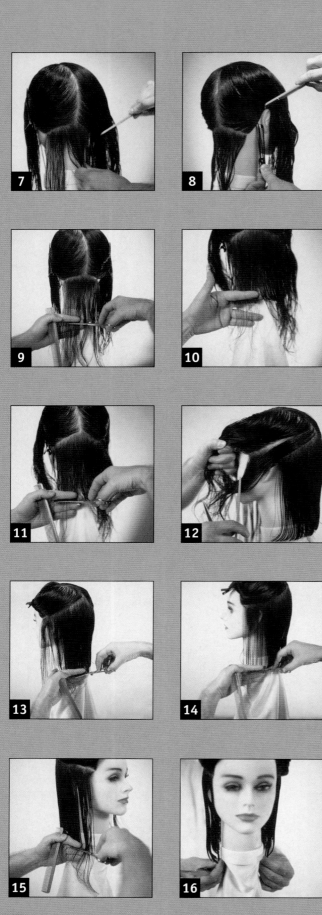

7. Starting on the left side of the nape, part off a 1/2" (1.25 cm) diagonal section from the center moving to below the ear.

8. Comb the remaining hair up and over the ear and clip in place. Repeat on the right side. Comb the remaining hair straight down. Notice how the diagonal lines for the part create an inverted V.

9. Hold the hair horizontally between the fingers of your left hand while holding the scissors horizontally in your right. With moderate tension, cut the left side, starting at the center and moving to the edge. Repeat on the right, cutting from the exterior to the center.

10. Release the next 1/2" (1.25 cm) section on both sides. You should be able to see the previously cut line—which is your cutting guide. Cut the section exactly on this guide.

11. Continue releasing 1/2" (1.25 cm) sections, cutting one side and then the other until you reach the crest. Maintain the diagonal partings and horizontal cutting position.

12. When you reach the point that is about 1/2" (1.25 cm) above the ear, take a diagonal part from the center back and bring it all the way through the entire side section to the front hairline on both sides.

13. Comb the section into natural fall. Begin cutting it from the back, moving toward the ear.

14. Continue cutting toward the front. Comb the hair into natural fall and cut horizontally.

15. Move to the opposite side and repeat the procedure.

16. Before proceeding, cross-check for balance by holding the two front side sections down and ensuring that they are the same length.

17. With the side length established, continue working up the side, bringing down 1/2" (1.25 cm) diagonally parted sections.

18. Cut the section to the established horizontal guideline. Complete the entire side up to the previously established part.

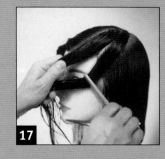 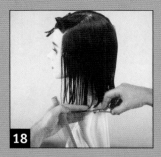

19. Once you have established the length, you can cut from front to back, using the previously cut sections as a guide. Continue bringing down 1/2" (1.25 cm) diagonal sections and cutting them.

20. When you reach the recession area at the corner of the eye, part out the front section.

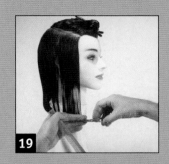 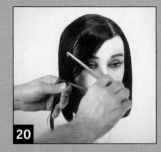

21. Clip the front section out of the way and continue cutting the side until it's complete.

22. Unclip the front section and comb it down neatly toward the side. Hold it to the side so that all the hair passes the eyebrow at the same point.

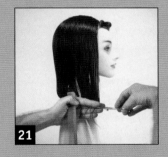 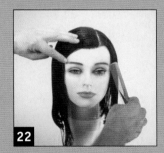

23. Hold the hair at the eyebrow with your fore-finger and comb the rest of the hair into natural fall.

24. Cut the hair in this position, using the side section as your guide. Check the nape length by directing the head forward and, if needed, cleaning up the line.

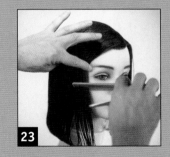 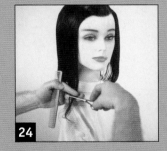

25. Apply the appropriate liquid styling formula before blow-drying into the sleek, blunt finish seen here.

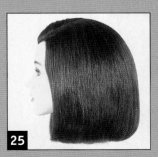

BLOW-DRYING HORIZONTAL BLUNT CUT

OVERVIEW

This style begins with the shoulder-length horizontal blunt cut. The style shown here will maintain and show off that classic cut; you'll use a blow-dryer and heat-resistant, rubber-based brush to create a full, even line. It is important that you take the time to section the head properly and to dry each section thoroughly with the brush and dryer. This will create a smooth shape that will highlight the exactness of the cut.

APPLY

With your clients, these technical steps will follow consultation, shampoo, and power or towel drying.

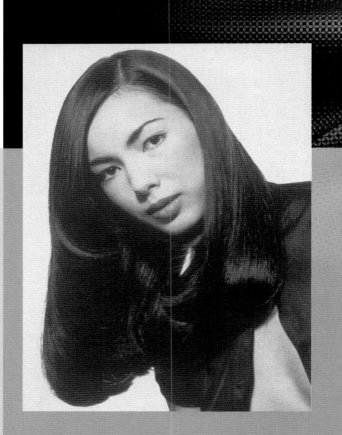

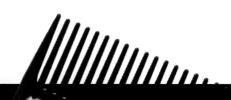

PROCEDURE

1. Towel dry, then power dry the hair to remove excess moisture. Apply a styling product of your choice and work it through the hair, paying particular attention to the base area.

2. Find the natural part in the hair, or determine the artificial part if this will be different from the hair's natural part. Section off the sides from the back—clip out of the way to control.

3. Divide the back into two sections by parting from ear to ear. Control and comb the top lengths and clip out of the way.

4. Beginning at the nape, use a heat-resistant, rubber-based brush to hold the hair initially at a low elevation. Follow the brush with a dryer at a medium setting while bending the ends in the preferred direction. Note how the nozzle of the blow-dryer is used when positioning hair lengths for brush work.

5., 6. Continue, using the same technique with 1" to 1 1/2" (2.5 to 3.75 cm) sections, up to the occipital area. Note the angle of the hair from the scalp when blow-drying—this accentuates the base lift.

7. Here you see the results developing on the back section—a smooth, rounded shape with a minimum of movement at the ends.

8. Continue with the style by subdividing the side section. Hold the hair at a low elevation with the brush and follow with the dryer, remembering to turn the edge of the brush to create a rounded edge or bend.

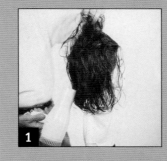
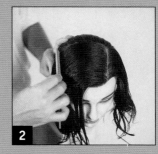
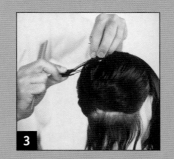
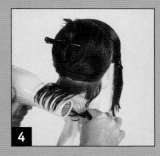
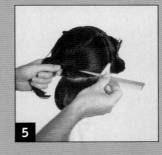
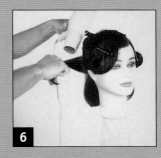
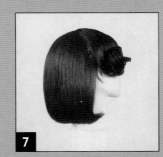
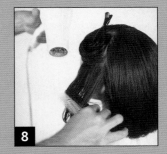

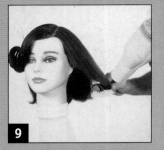

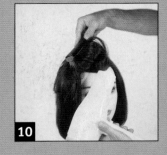

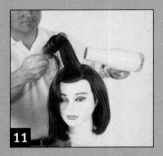

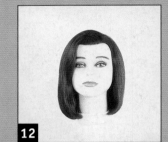

9. Continue in the same way through the rest of the side section. Turn the brush through the ends to accentuate roundness.

10. Starting with the front section, hold the hair straight up from the head. Dry the base or scalp area of the hair. At the fringe area, push the hair into a curvature shape, drying a wave formation into place. As the wave begins to form, roll the brush back to encourage a deeper wave. Work through the top with vertical sections.

11. Next, work through the top as shown. Continue drying from mid-shaft to the hair ends in the manner as outlined.

12. The finished style shows smooth, sleek lines that accentuate the horizontal blunt cut.

They can because they think they can.

Virgil

CREATE

Apply this technique to different lengths, colors, and textures for almost endless possibilities.

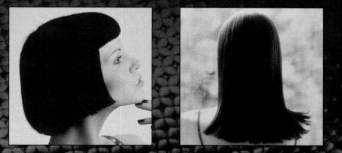

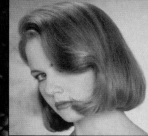

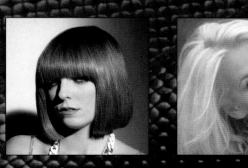

DIAGONAL FORWARD BLUNT

OVERVIEW

A true classic, this cut was first introduced in the Sassoon salon and was later referred to as the A-line or bias-line. The dynamic diagonal line gives it a swingy, free-moving quality. It's cut shorter at the center back area, then lengthens as it travels to the front. The shorter hair will push and direct the longer hair, making the A-line cut move forward. The side parting makes for an evocative and dramatic sweep of hair as it frames the face.

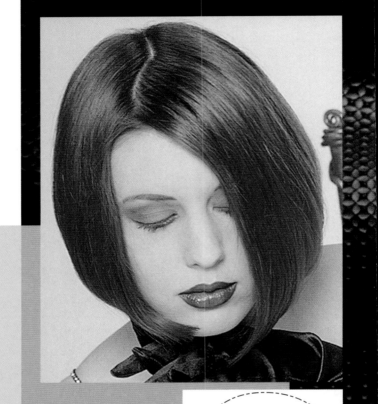

APPLY

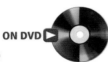 ON DVD ▶

With your clients, these technical steps will follow the consultation and shampoo.

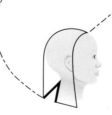

In the diagonal forward blunt cut, lengths progress from the exterior area to the interior. All lengths fall to one level along the forward diagonal perimeter frame.

PROCEDURE

1. Establish a side part and gently comb the hair into place with the head held upright. Comb all the hair in natural fall. Make certain the ends are combed neatly in place.

2. Part the back from the crown straight down to the nape, dividing it into two equal sections.

3. Take a 1/2" (1.25 cm) diagonal parting from the center to the ear and comb it down.

4. Clip the remaining hair out of the way and repeat on the opposite side. Begin cutting on the left side. Comb the section down. Holding the hair straight down with the back of your hand, angle your fingers from the center of the back to create a diagonal forward line. Maintain moderate tension as you cut against the neck, along the bottom of your little finger.

5. Move to the right side. Comb the hair down and place your hand so that it forms a diagonal forward line. Standing just to the left of this section to allow for comfort, hold the hair with your left hand and cut with your right. Using consistent tension, cut against the neck from the center to the side. Notice that the scissors are held palm up.

6. Return to the left side. Continue to bring down 1/2" (1.25 cm) diagonal sections from both sides and cut to match the length and angle of the previously cut section.

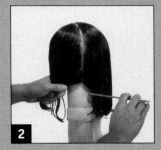
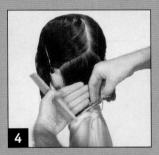
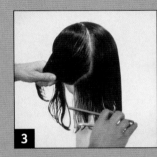
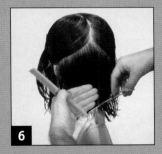
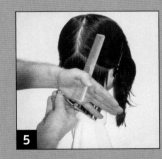
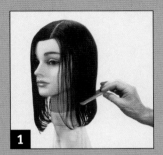

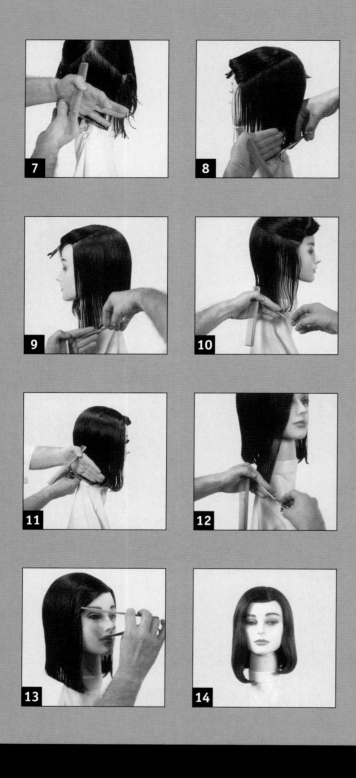

7. Repeat the procedure on the right side, again cutting the new 1/2" (1.25 cm) section to your established guide. When you move from the left to the right side, switch from holding your scissors palm down to palm up.

8. Continue in this manner until you reach the crest. Standing in front of your mannequin, take a diagonal parting that moves all the way from the center back, through the side, to the front. With the head straight up, comb the sides and back in natural fall and continue diagonal cutting from the center back toward the front.

9. When you reach the ear, move toward the side. Holding the hair between your index and middle fingers, complete the diagonal forward line by bringing down subsequent 1/2" (1.25 cm) sections until the entire side is cut.

10. Move to the opposite side and repeat the procedure, bringing down 1/2" (1.25 cm) sections and cutting to establish the diagonal forward side lengths. Move the head forward as you cut the back area against the skin. Position the head upright as you cut the side area between the fingers along the diagonal forward line.

11. Continue bringing down sections until you reach the recession area up from the outside corner of the eye. At this point, section out the top front area, clip it out of the way, and complete the right side, bringing down 1/2" (1.25 cm) sections and cutting them along the established diagonal forward line.

12. With both sides complete, bring down the front section, comb it in natural fall, and cut it diagonally to blend with the already established line.

13. To check the line of the cut, push the heavy right side back at the eyebrow to match the hair combed into this position on the opposite side. Check the lengths for balance. Refine the line, if necessary.

14. The finished cut exhibits a gentle diagonal perimeter line around the face. The weight line provides for great freedom of movement.

The journey of a thousand miles begins with a single step.

Chinese Proverb

OVERVIEW

This style begins with the diagonal forward blunt cut. As when you styled the horizontal blunt cut, you'll maintain the neat lines of the classic blunt cut while directing more hair forward, toward the face. It's a classic look with a contemporary twist that will work for a variety of clients' face shapes, ages, and lifestyles.

APPLY

With your clients, these technical steps will follow consultation, shampoo, and power or towel drying.

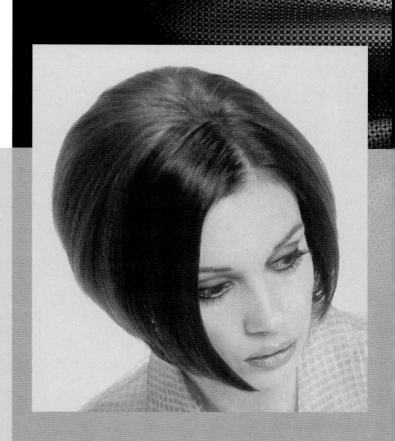

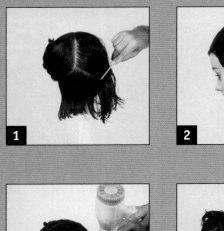

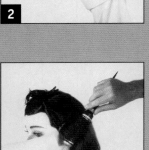

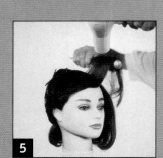

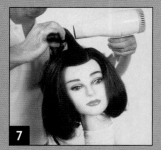

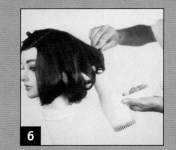

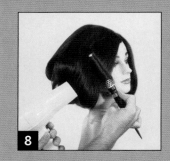

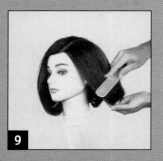

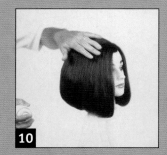

PROCEDURE

1. Part the hair from the top of the ear, over the top of the head, to the other ear. Subdivide the back section, first down the center back, then the nape area. Part off diagonally on either side, then comb and clip the upper lengths out of the way.

2. Starting at the nape and using a round brush, roll the hair over the brush and raise and lower the brush while following it with a dryer.

3. Continue this procedure up the back area in 1" to 1 1/2" (2.5 cm to 3.75 cm) sections. Revolve the round brush along the lengths of the hair to create the end fullness. Use tension for the ultimate smoothing effect.

4. Continue through to the side section starting with the section over the ear, then moving up toward the side part.

5. At the side part area, hold the section straight out while you dry the base area, and continue through to the ends.

6. Switch to a smaller brush and redefine the ends by first adding heat, then pressing the cooling button. Continue through the perimeter area following the lines of the cut. This will give a tremendous amount of extra fullness on the ends.

7. To create more height in the top area, hold the hair straight out from the base. First dry the base, then continue outward through the hair lengths for added strength.

8. To create a flipped-under effect, roll the hair toward the face while drying, then cooling, from underneath (for added strength).

9. Again, use a small brush to accentuate the ends. Brush and loosen the entire design.

10. To finish the design, spray the top surface of the hair, and smooth with your hand. The diagonal forward blunt cut with swingy voluminous movement—a modern classic!

Genius is 99 percent perspiration and 1 percent inspiration.

Thomas Edison

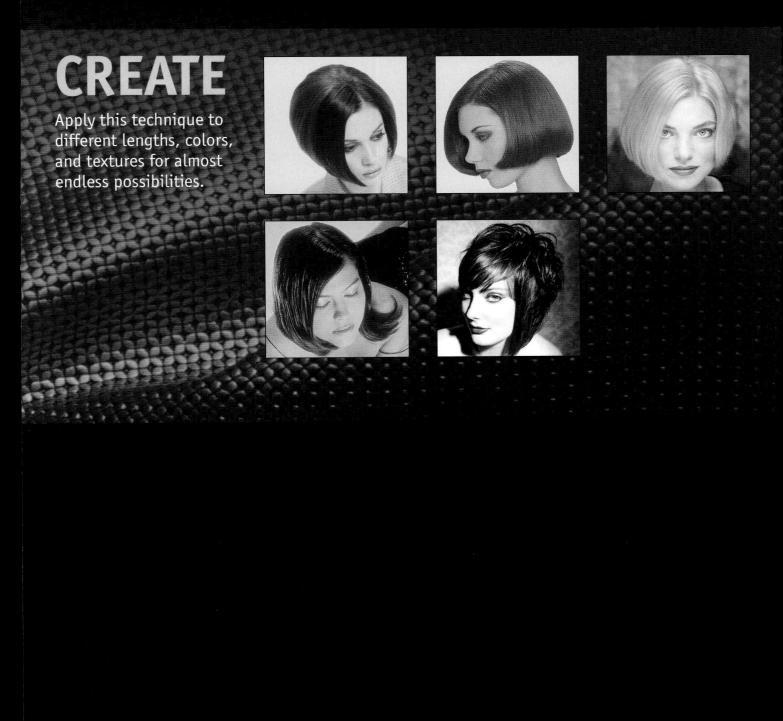

CREATE

Apply this technique to different lengths, colors, and textures for almost endless possibilities.

DIAGONAL BACK BLUNT

OVERVIEW

The diagonal back blunt cut has a curvy, continuous perimeter line, creating a fluid look. Shorter at the front, then lengthening at the center back, this style—also called a pageboy—provides much versatility in its styling options. The line allows for great freedom of movement, perhaps one reason why Sassoon chose this cut—originally created for the famous dancer Isadora Duncan—to reinterpret. This shorter version of the "Isadora" cut is indeed poetry in motion.

APPLY

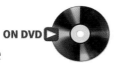

With your clients, these technical steps will follow the consultation and shampoo.

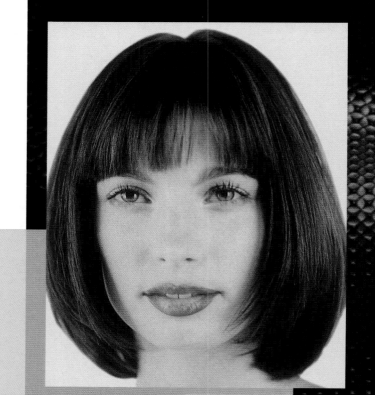

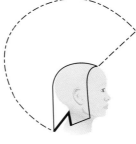

The diagonal back frame moves from just below the jaw to the collar area at the back of the head.

PROCEDURE

1. Prepare for this cut by parting as in the previous blunt cut. On the left side, position the back of your hand against the head so your fingers point down toward the nape and your wrist is slightly elevated. Hold both hands left of the center of your body. Using a palm-down cutting position, cut diagonally from the center back to the side.

2. For the right side, use the palm-up cutting position. Angle your hand by dropping your wrist, with fingers pointing toward the ear. Both hands are to the right of the center of your body. Cut from the center back toward the side.

3. Return to the left side, part off another 1/2" (1.25 cm) diagonal section of hair, and cut, moving your hands to the left of the center of your body and using the palm-down cutting position. The fingertips of the hand holding the hair should angle downward, elevating the wrist slightly.

4. Continue moving side to side and cutting 1/2" (1.25 cm) diagonal sections up to the crest. Maintain 0-degree elevation, even tension, and the diagonal back cutting line.

5. When you reach the crest, take a 1/2" (1.25 cm) diagonal parting that moves all the way from the center back, through the side, to the front. With the head straight up, comb the sides and back in natural fall. Cut the side section, using your hand to continue the diagonal back line from the back section you just cut to the front.

6. As you reach the front, move your body into position at the side. Bring down subsequent sections and complete the left side.

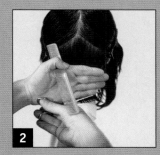

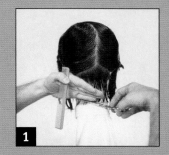

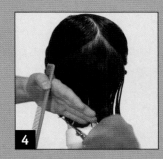

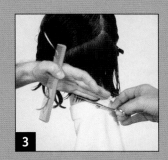

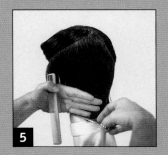

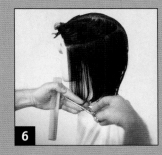

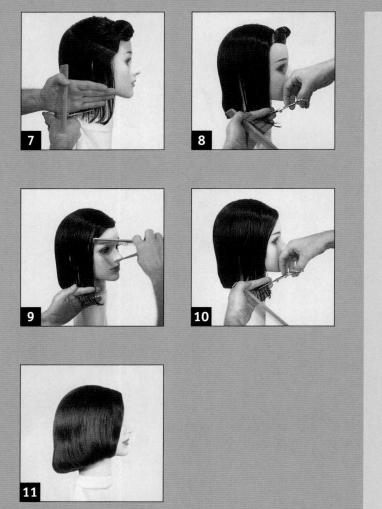

7. Move to the right side. Take a parting from the back through the side, and cut. Use 0-degree elevation and position your hand to continue the diagonal back line.

8. When you reach the recession area at the corner of the eye, clip the front fringe out of the way and complete cutting the right side.

9. Check the cut for balance, making certain both sides are cut to the same length at the same angle. Release the front fringe and comb it down. Push the heavy right side back at the eyebrow to match the position of the hair on the opposite side.

10. Holding the front section and the side guide together, cut the front section.

11. In the finished cut, the strong diagonal back line is evident.

Success is the sum of small efforts, repeated day in and day out.

Robert Collier

OVERVIEW

One of the most requested services in the salon is blow-drying hair with texture into a straight shape. This style is relatively easy—but it takes patience, the right tools, and the right styling products. Focusing on one section at a time is the key to a straight finished design.

APPLY

With your clients, these technical steps will follow consultation, shampoo, and power or towel drying.

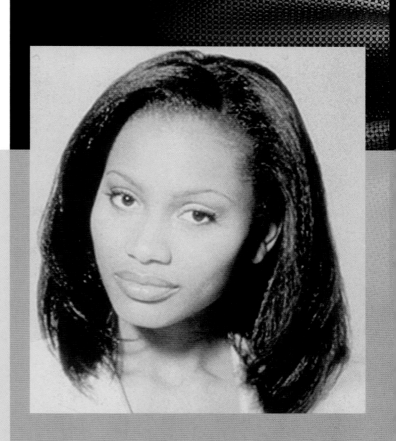

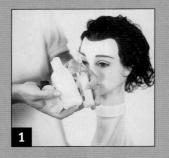

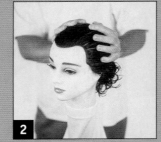

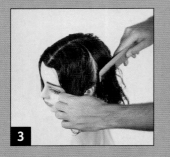

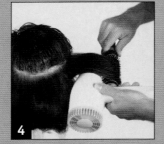

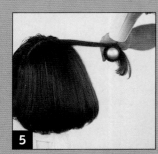

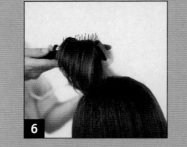

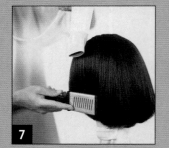

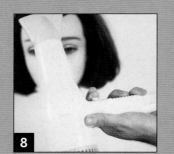

PROCEDURE

1. Some of the styling products you can choose from are liquid gel, conditioning foam, and silicone shiner. You may even choose to combine them.

2. Apply the product of your choice and work it through the hair.

3. The hair will be divided into 1" (2.5 cm) sections throughout the entire head for blow-drying. Clip the upper hair neatly out of the way. Start drying at the nape area. Use a large, round bristled brush to stretch and dry the hair. This type of brush allows for extra tension.

4. Use the side of the nozzle to maintain control of the section you're drying. This nozzle is inserted under the strand of hair to hold in place when repositioning the brush.

5. Follow the round brush with the dryer. Keep the brush and air flow moving through the hair.

6. Use tension to stretch the top surface of the hair for a smoother finish. Move the heat over the surface of the hair more slowly than normal, because it takes more heat to straighten.

7. Holding the hair tightly, add heat to the surface of the finished style.

8. Use the cooling button on the blow-dryer to help set in movement or smoothness.

9. Use the curve of the brush to add bend to the ends of the hair.

10. Smooth the hair with a wide-toothed comb. Lightly spray the shape for hold or work a shiner product through the top surface.

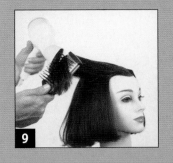

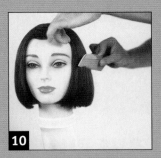

11. The finished style has a smooth texture, which defines the diagonal back blunt shape. Curly hair has been transformed through the blow-drying technique.

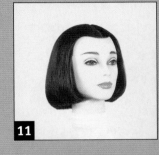

It is better to light a candle than curse the darkness.

Chinese Proverb

CREATE

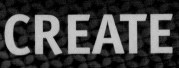

Apply this technique to different lengths, colors, and textures for almost endless possibilities.

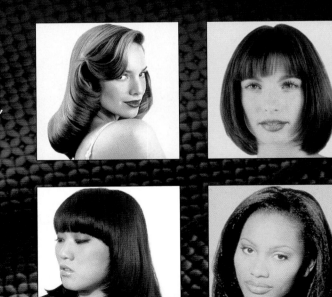

BLUNT CUT ON DRY HAIR

OVERVIEW

Time management is a top priority for today's hectic pace of living. A good time management technique for your clients with very curly hair is to invest more time in chemical relaxer services, conditioning treatments, and preparation of the hair by blow-drying smooth (pre-prep) before you begin cutting and finishing.

Hair that is highly textured (curly, for instance) appears completely different when wet. When this kind of hair dries, it contracts in length as the curl pulls it up. Cutting hair of this type dry gives you more control over the creation of the shape. Once the hair is relaxed to be straight and smooth, an unlimited variety of sculpted styles can be created from this foundation.

The dry cutting technique is a classic, condensed cutting and finishing concept.

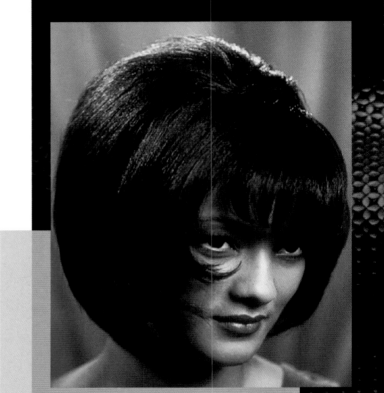

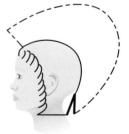

Pre-existing internal layers flow over the perimeter blunt weight line. The notched areas around the front hairline are cut bluntly.

APPLY

ON DVD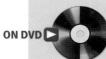

With your clients, these technical steps will follow the consultation. The relaxer treatment is performed first, followed by the conditioning and color treatments.

To prepare for the cut, blow-dry the hair smoothly.

PROCEDURE

1. After blow-drying, use a dry wrapping technique to straighten, control, and smooth the hair for dry cutting. Brush or comb all the dry hair around the head, then blow-dry for a few minutes or put under a warm dryer to "set" the wrapped hair direction.

2. This will create natural-looking curved movement, with the hair contouring close to the head shape, a result that is not generally achieved by chemically relaxing, blow-drying, or ironing hair.

3. Now the hair is ready for a dry designer cut.

4. Brush the hair in the direction of the desired cut.

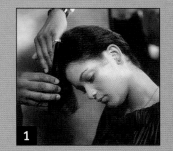
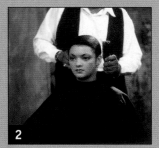
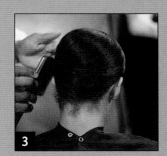
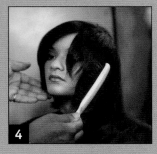

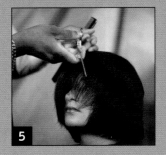

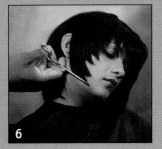

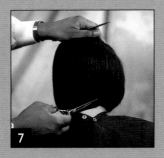

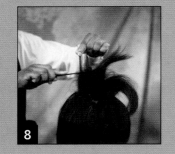

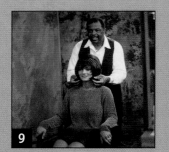

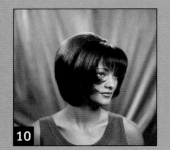

5. Diagonally blunt cut a line over the left eye. You will do notching on either side of this line. This technique is free-form in nature—you are notching into the lengths around the front hairline at measured, slightly irregular intervals.

6. After completing the fringe area, move to the right side. Continue to create your design around the face using the notching technique. Repeat on the left side.

7. After completing the left and right sides, move to the back section. Create a blunt weight line at the desired length.

8. Backcomb the hair on the top of the head to create a base for volume through the crown area. Smooth and curl the hair. You have an entire head of hair that is consistent in texture, with soft curls for movement.

9. Spray the hair for hold. Spray on fingers and detail around the face. The client's makeover is complete. Her hair has been transformed!

10. The consistent texture and soft movement complement the closely contoured blunt shape, results that are accentuated through the dry wrapping and cutting techniques. The finished style is progressively classic, with hair that is shiny and silky.

GRADUATED BLUNT

OVERVIEW

In this cut you will combine two distinctively different shapes in a harmonious fashion. The graduated nape area flows into a blunt diagonal forward shape toward the front and sides of the design. To create the cut, you will learn two new techniques: the use of graduation through the nape area and the use of pointing to refine the graduation as well as the perimeter line. This graduated blunt cut—some call it the graduated bob—is modern in its silhouette, and its diagonal forward line gives great freedom of movement. The close-fitting nape area is very sculptural in nature, while the rest of the cut features great structure and shape.

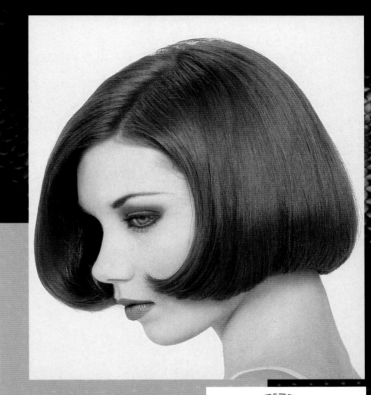

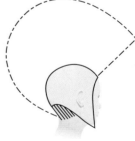

The graduated blunt cut is a modern classic. The sculpted graduation at the nape falls into a beautifully defined weight area at the sides.

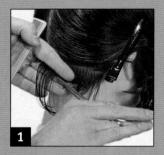

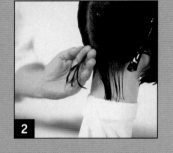

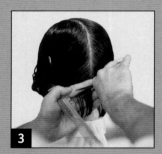

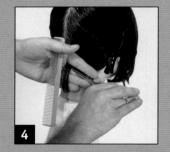

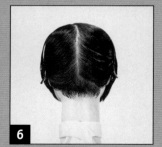

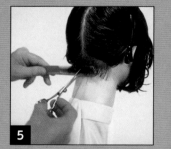

APPLY

ON DVD ▶

With your clients, these technical steps will follow the consultation and shampoo.

PROCEDURE

1. In this cut we'll use the palm-to-palm scissor position.

2. Preparing the hair as in blunt haircutting, begin cutting in the back on the left side. Comb and elevate the hair, holding it one finger's distance from the base area. This is a one-finger elevation or holding position for creating graduation.

3. Cut the section diagonally along the inside of the middle finger of your left hand, which is holding the hair. Notice how the entire left hand is angled downward to the left.

4. Repeat the procedure on the right side, cutting the hair in the opposite direction.

5. To refine the perimeter shape at the nape, hold the section out with your comb and use a pointing technique.

6. When complete, the first section already shows graduation: Rather than lying flat, the hair stacks along the graduated angle you have cut.

7. Release the next 1/2" (1.25 cm) section. You should be able to see the previously cut guide through it.

8. Comb the hair down and out at a medium elevation and cut, following the established guideline.

9. Repeat this procedure on the opposite side.

10. Continue to bring down 1/2" (1.25 cm) sections and cut to your guide. This will be the procedure as you work up the back area. Do not shift the hair away from the natural fall direction.

11. When you reach the crest, you will begin to work on the sides.

12. Part all the way through the sides, taking a diagonal forward section that's no more than 1/2" (1.25 cm) over the ear. Bring the head upright. Cut diagonally with a low holding position. Position your fingers to establish the length and create the diagonal line; cut the entire side section, holding the hair as close to the skin as possible.

13. Comb the hair against the skin and check the line for accuracy. This will accentuate a blunt line.

14. Move to the opposite side. Bring down a 1/2" (1.25 cm) diagonal parting over the ear. Bring the head upright. Holding the hair low, begin cutting at the graduated back. Cut diagonally forward with the hair in natural fall. Position your fingers to establish the length and create the diagonal line; cut the entire side section, working as close to the skin as possible.

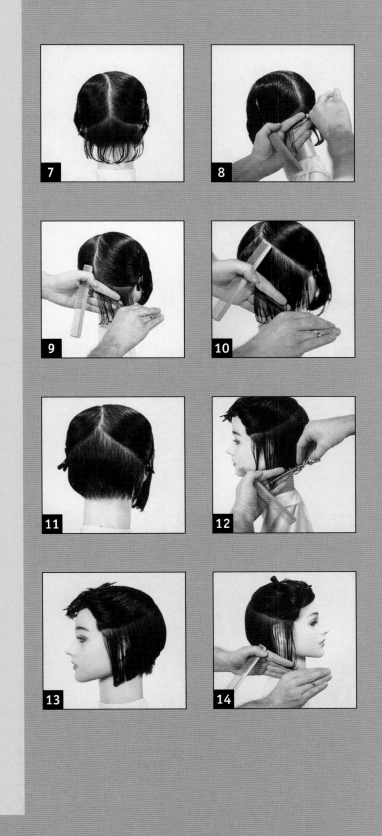

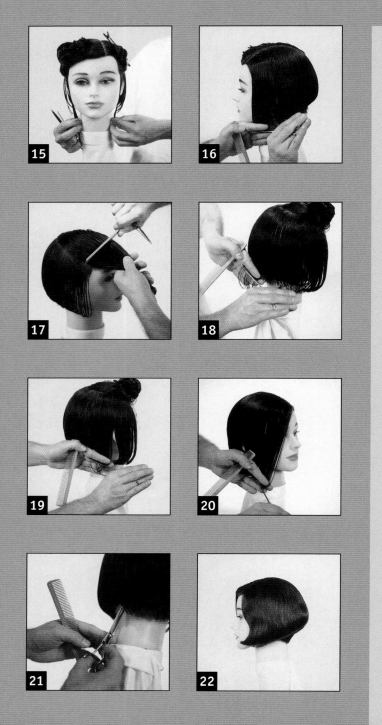

15. Before cutting subsequent partings at the sides, check the lengths on both sides to make certain they are even.

16. Return to the left side. Part out diagonally, releasing 1/2" (1.25 cm) sections. Cut, following the established guideline. Maintain the natural fall direction when working toward the sides, holding the hair as low as possible. Continue to use this technique to the top side parting.

17. Continue on the right side, parting out diagonally to release sections.

18. Maintain natural fall while cutting through the sides, following the established guide. Continue to follow the established guideline to cut diagonally toward the front and sides.

19. Move to the side and cut in natural fall.

20. Section out the top front fringe area, comb it to the heavy right side, and cut it at an angle through the front that blends with the sides. Cutting of the top is performed on the heavy side of the part—the right side—only.

21. Check the entire perimeter using the pointing technique.

22. The sculptural silhouette seen here is a magnificent shape to be adapted in a variety of ways. The precision of the shape gives the style a modern appeal.

Tough times never last, but tough people do.

BLOW-DRYING GRADUATED BLUNT

OVERVIEW

This style begins with the graduated blunt cut that you completed in the haircutting part of the program. Styling this cut with an asymmetric look is very slimming to the face and answers the needs of the client who wants to move her hair off her face. Again, the simple movement of the brush and blow-dryer through the hair will create body and ornamental effects without diminishing the sculptural silhouette of the cut.

APPLY

With your clients, these technical steps will follow consultation, shampoo, and power or towel drying.

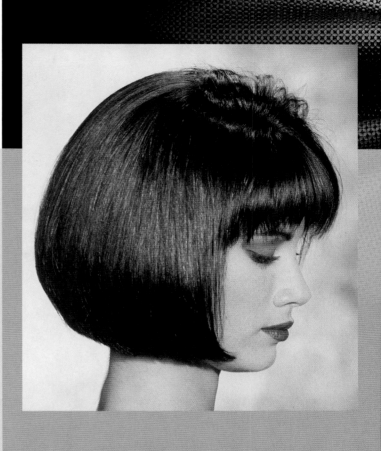

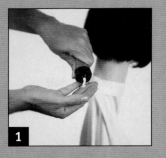

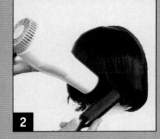

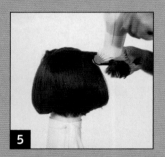

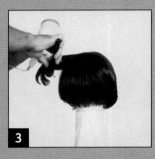

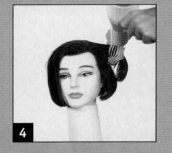

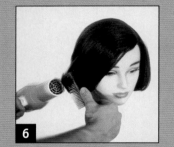

PROCEDURE

1. Apply a styling product of your choice, and work it through the hair. Use a side part as a design part.

2. Begin contouring in the nape area with the rubber-based bristle brush. Directionally flow the hair outward from the center back on either side. The air flow follows the brush as it closely contours the hair against the head.

3. Above the occipital area, begin parting out along a diagonal forward. Insert the last two rows of the brush to lift and direct the hair while blow-drying. Continue upward and maintain the brush while drying along the diagonal forward.

4. Continue this process into the sides and up to the side part. Lift the hair out from the base area according to the amount of base lift desired. Turn the ends and dry to bevel the ends under.

5. Repeat the process on the other side of the head. Concentrate on using precise blow-drying technique. Alternate the brush through the lengths and bevel the ends for a rounded weight line.

6. Finish blow-drying the front area, paying particular attention to the base area and mid-shaft. The ends will be dried upward. Grasp the ends in the brush and turn upward to create a flipped effect.

CREATE

Apply this technique to different lengths, colors, and textures for almost endless possibilities.

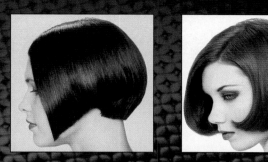

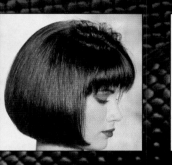

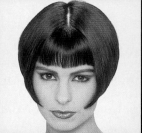

LOW GRADUATION

OVERVIEW

In this classic graduated shape, lengths flow diagonally back away from the face. This mid-length style is perfect for the client who likes the look of long hair but appreciates the control and manageability of a short cut.

After you create the graduated shape, you will soften the edges of the graduated weight line by removing the weight corner. This will modernize the shape and create softly rounded edges.

APPLY

ON DVD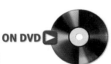

With your clients, these technical steps will follow the consultation and shampoo.

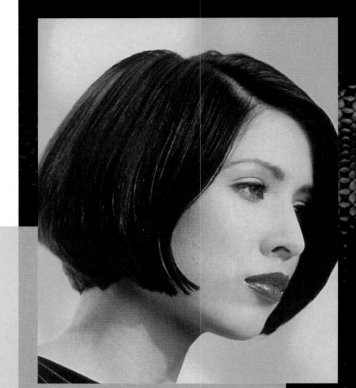

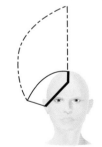

This very popular, commercial style features a graduated frame that flows back off the face. The mid-length shape features a line that travels from the tip of the nose to approximately one inch below the nape area in the back.

PROCEDURE

1. Establish a side part, combing the hair into natural fall with the head upright. Make sure the ends are neatly combed. Working off a side part, comb the hair back over the ear. Diagonally part a 1/2" (1.25 cm) section just in front of the ear, moving from the front hairline back over the ear.

2. Use a low (one-finger) elevation. Angle the fingers holding the hair from the tip of the nose to the ear lobe. Use the palm-to-palm scissor position as you cut.

3. This diagonally angled line will be your cutting guide. Notice that it angles from the nose to the ear lobe.

4. Part off the next section, angling down from the hairline to the back, so the part line falls 1/2" (1.25 cm) above the top of the ear. Comb the hair into the natural fall direction and cut on the diagonal, following the established guide.

5. Hold your scissors low in a palm-to-palm position. Taking care not to cut past your second knuckle, extend the guide through to the back.

6. Continue bringing down 1/2" (1.25 cm) sections and cutting to the previous guide. (Make certain you can see the guide through each new section.) Cut exactly on your guide.

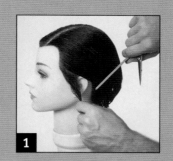
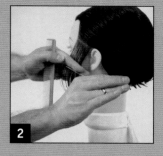
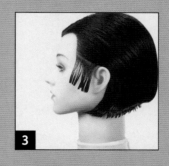
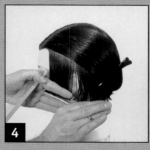
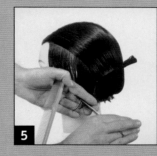
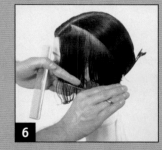

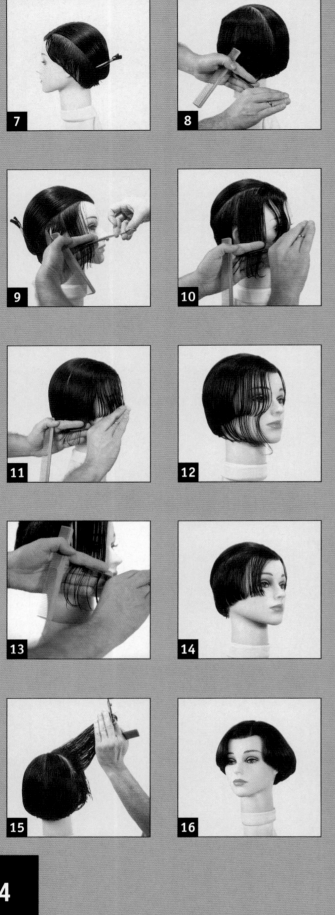

7. The completed sections should form a perfect diagonal line from front to back.

8. Complete the entire side, diagonally parting out 1/2" (1.25 cm) sections and following the guide. Maintain the low one-finger elevation. Comb the lengths against the skin and refine the perimeter line. Comb the line between the fingers and point in to blend and refine the back area.

9., 10. Move to the opposite side. Establish a guide as described in step 3. Cut subsequent sections as in steps 5 through 8 until you reach the recession area.

11. Part through from the center front hairline. Notice that the front hairline is left out. Cut through from the side to the nape. Blend and cut the fringe in natural fall. The horizontal finger position is aligned with the tip of the nose. Continue working upward using this procedure. Cut the sides to the guide, then cut the fringe to the guide. Remember to use the natural fall direction and low elevation.

12. Comb all the top hair and front fringe down in the natural fall direction. Here you can see the guide through the final, front section.

13. Cut the fringe line to adapt to the needs and desires of your client.

14. The completed side shows that the front piece extends toward the tip of the nose.

15. If you wish to soften the weight line by removing the corner, work radially through the interior, bringing sections up and out and taking the weight corner off. You can do this blunt, pointed, or notched in.

16. The graduated diagonal back silhouette flows into a softly rounded back area. The weight area, having been rounded, creates a soft shape.

BLOW-DRYING LOW GRADUATION

OVERVIEW

This style begins with the low graduation, mid-length cut you completed in the haircutting part of the program. The use of radial sections through the interior of the head makes the blow-drying of graduated shapes fast, easy, and efficient. You'll use both the round and paddle brushes to get the most volume for this style.

APPLY

With your clients, these technical steps will follow consultation, shampoo, and power or towel drying.

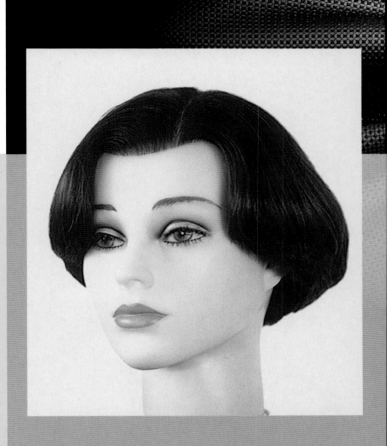

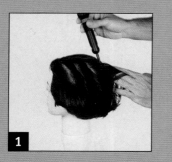

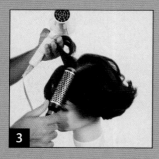

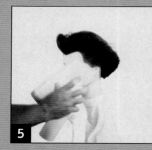

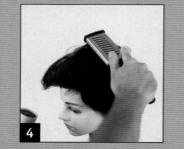

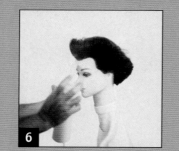

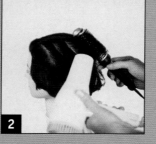

PROCEDURE

1. Apply a styling product of your choice, and work it through the hair. Use a round brush to part the hair into diagonal sections through the interior.

2. Work around the head using the dryer to follow the round brush positioned diagonally.

3. In the top area, direct lengths forward, then roll toward the base as blow-drying. This will maximize volume given the over-directed base. Continue this technique toward the front hairline area. The front fringe section is rolled using the same technique to create a volume effect in this area.

4. Use a paddle airflow brush to stretch the shape and brush into place.

5. Use a hair spray and dryer technique to finish the design. Spray directionally up and into the front hairline lengths while following with the blow-dryer. This will create enhanced directional hold, body, and lift. Again, brush through with the large paddle brush to loosen the lines of the style.

6. The finished style is very commercial and wearable for a large number of clientele. The technique may be adapted on a variety of other haircuts.

CREATE

Apply this technique to different lengths, colors, and textures for almost endless possibilities.

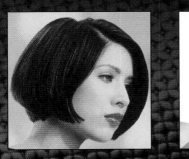
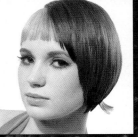
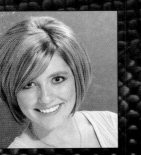
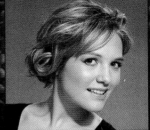

HORIZONTAL GRADUATION

OVERVIEW

In this silhouette, a uniquely geometric front and sides contrast to the highly graduated nape area. This short, contoured nape harmonizes beautifully with the low graduation cut horizontally at the front of the design.

APPLY

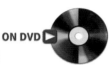 ON DVD

With your clients, these technical steps will follow the consultation and shampoo.

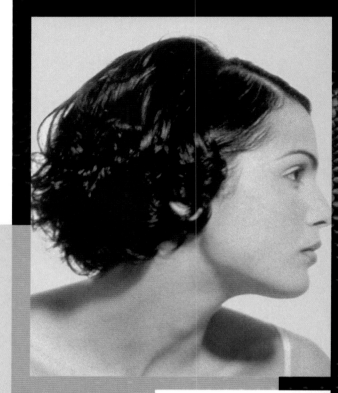

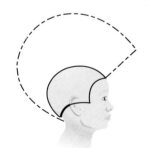

This short, exacting cut may be styled back off the face to accentuate the flow of graduation. This is an easy-care, easy-wear shape given the precise lines of the graduated shape. Horizontal lines at the sides move into the diagonally graduated back.

PROCEDURE

1. Establish a side part, combing the hair into natural fall with the head upright. Make sure the ends are neatly combed. Part the back from the crown straight down to the nape, dividing it into two equal sections. After establishing a side part, comb the hair on the left side over the ear. Diagonally part out a 1/2″ (1.25 cm) section in front of the ear, comb it in natural fall, and establish the length, using a horizontal cutting position and low elevation holding position.

2. Release the next diagonal back section and cut to the horizontal guide, holding in low elevation.

3. Diagonally part another 1/2″ (1.25 cm) section from the front hairline to the nape, following the perimeter hairline. Cut the side horizontally to the established guideline using low elevation. Continue the line behind the ear diagonally, using low elevation. The hair through the back is shifted out of natural fall toward the diagonal guideline created behind the ear.

4. Cut the entire section behind the ear to the nape in this manner.

5. Bring down the next 1/2″ (1.25 cm) diagonal section from the front hairline to the nape. Comb the hair neatly into natural fall. Cut the side horizontally, using low elevation. You're beginning to build graduation.

6. Angle your fingers down toward the nape to blend the back of this section into the diagonal back guide and continue cutting, using a medium elevation with the traveling guide.

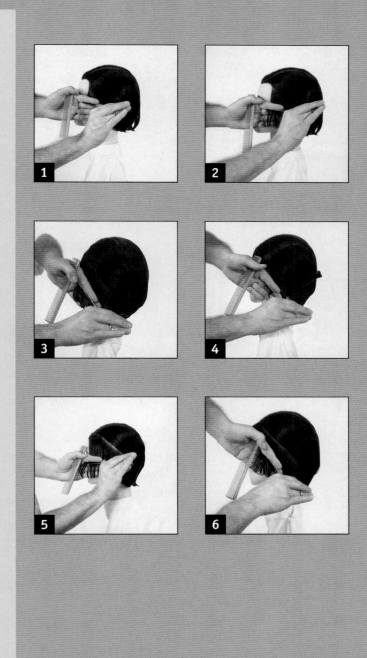

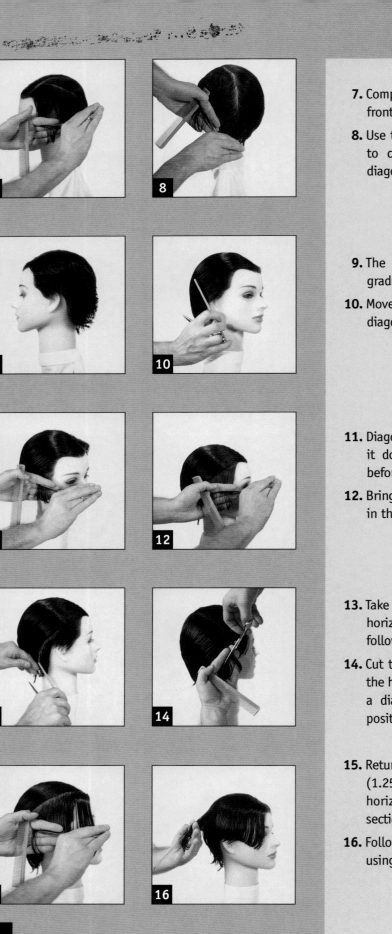

7. Complete the entire side, cutting the section in front of the ear horizontally.

8. Use the traveling guide with medium elevation to continue cutting the back section on a diagonal.

9. The completed left side shows activated graduation.

10. Move to the right side and comb the hair diagonally toward the back.

11. Diagonally part a 1/2" (1.25 cm) section, comb it down, and cut it horizontally, as you did before, using low elevation.

12. Bring down a second diagonal parting and cut it in the same manner.

13. Take a diagonal parting from just above the horizontally cut sections all the way to the nape, following the hairline.

14. Cut the side. Then, starting at the back end of the horizontal guide, cut the back section along a diagonal, using the low elevation holding position.

15. Return to the front. Bring down another 1/2" (1.25 cm) diagonal section. Cut the side area horizontally, leaving out the front fringe section.

16. Follow this section into the area behind the ear, using a traveling guide with medium elevation.

17. Continue to graduate the lengths along a diagonal line until you reach the center back.

18. Direct the front piece that you left out toward the side. Cut the front piece at an extreme angle toward the lip line.

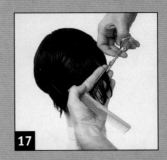
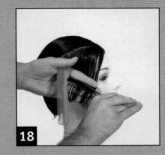

19. Continue working to the top using the techniques as outlined. Continue into the back area using consistent holding, cutting, and scissor positions as established. Check both sides at the center back by combing the hair straight out.

20. As a final step, check upward horizontally through the center back.

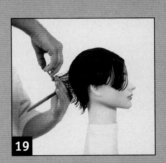
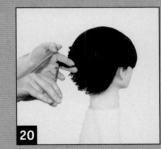

21. The finished cut is styled in its natural flow and direction to highlight the horizontally cut front. There is a subtle asymmetry at the frame area. The hair styled back off the face accentuates the graduated effect. A slight graduation around the sides flows into a more highly graduated back area that contours to the curve of the head.

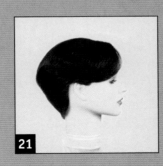

OVERVIEW

This style begins with the graduated, short-length horizontal cut you completed in the haircutting part of this program. As with the mid-length, graduated style, the keys to creating body and movement are the use of the round brush and your blow-drying technique. Because of the shorter hair length, you'll use a large-tooth comb and your fingers to stretch the hair in front; this adds an interesting contrast to the tapered back.

APPLY

With your clients, these technical steps will follow consultation, shampoo, and power or towel drying.

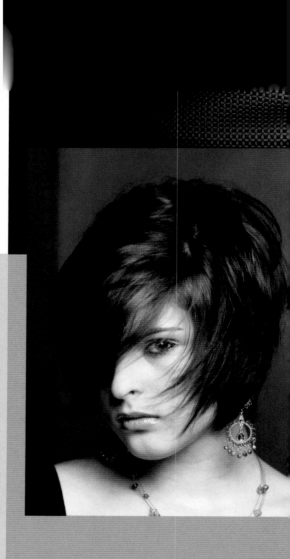

PROCEDURE

1. Apply a styling product of your choice.

2. Work the product through the hair.

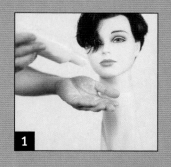

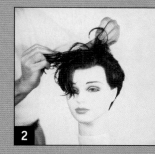

3. Begin to dry the hair in the nape area, using a brush to direct and shape the hair.

4. Using a round metal brush, roll sections of hair in the back of the crown and blow-dry. A one-diameter base area (to the size of the brush) is rolled to position on base for perfect volume.

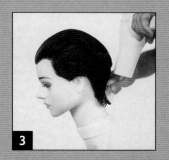

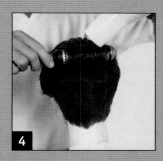

5. Move forward in the crown area, one section at a time, using a one-diameter on-base technique. The hair is held 45 degrees from the center of the base and rolled.

6. Secure the rolled hair with long clips at the scalp.

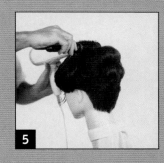

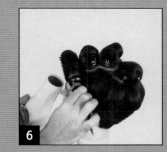

7. Continue to blow-dry rolled sections, working toward the front hairline area. Clip each section as completed.

8. Remove the clips through the interior. Complete the side section by connecting the side hairline lengths with the front fringe area. Lightly spray while directing the airflow.

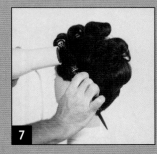

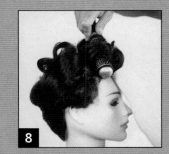

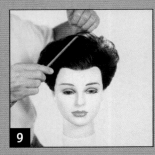

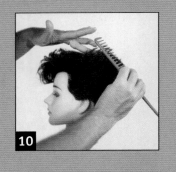

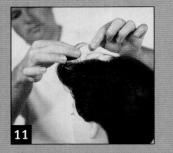

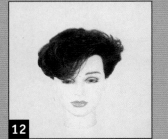

9., 10. Comb through the set with a texture comb to blend and shape the hair.

11. Use your fingers to place and style the ends. Continue to place the hair into the style lines. Lightly spray.

12. The finished style features lift and movement in the crown with a softly directed fringe.

CREATE

Apply this technique to different lengths, colors, and textures for almost endless possibilities.

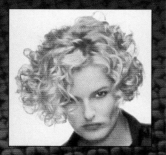
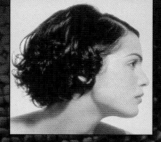
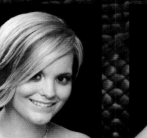
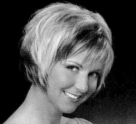

LAYERED SQUARE SHAPE

OVERVIEW

This dynamic short shape will provide your client with a silhouette that features weight emphasis and length to frame the face and add volume to the back of the head. The shape is more closely contoured or layered above the ears and through the top area of the head. It's a very wearable, distinctive geometric shape that can be styled in a variety of ways—ideal for the client who likes to wear her hair short or for the client who may have a less-than-perfect head shape. You'll revisit this cut again and again.

When performing this cut on a client in its entirety, you would first cut the perimeter frame along the desired lines either as a blunt or graduated shape.

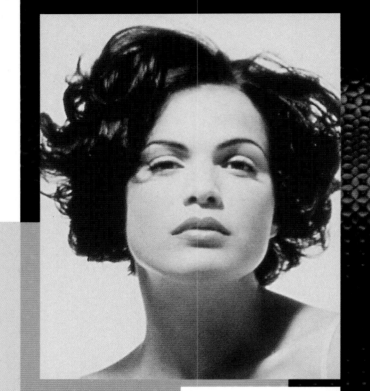

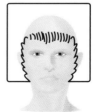

Shown here is the finished layered shape. The weight areas within this haircut emphasize a unique dimension. This haircut is suitable for a wide range of clients.

APPLY

ON DVD ▶

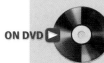

With your clients, these technical steps will follow the consultation and shampoo.

PROCEDURE

1. First, comb the hair in natural fall. Establish a center part.

2. Part out a 1/2" (1.25 cm) vertical section from behind the ear to establish a guide. Comb this hair straight out from the side of the head into a horizontal holding position. In this cut, the guide will be approximately 3" (7.5 cm), out from the ear area.

3. Cut this section along a vertical line.

4. Bring the front area, in 1/2" (1.25 cm) sections back to the guide.

5. Notice that while you're holding the hair straight out from the side, the cutting position is vertical. Notice that the scissor position is also vertical.

6. Bring sections from the back forward to this guide and cut, using 1/2" (1.25 cm) sections. Work all the way to the center back with sections that pivot around the crown.

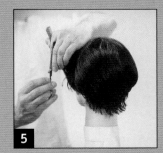

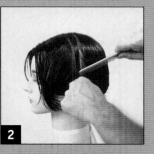

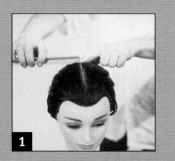

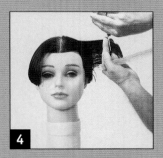

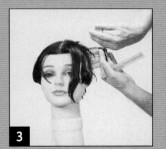

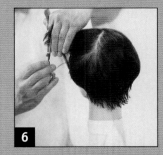

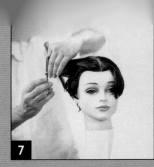

7.

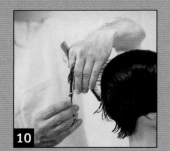

7. Repeat the procedure outlined for the side area, bringing 1/2" (1.25 cm) sections from the top and sides back to the guide at the ear and then cutting.

8. Take a 1/2" (1.25 cm) vertical section from directly behind the ear and cut to the guide.

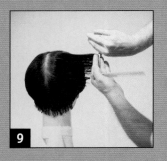

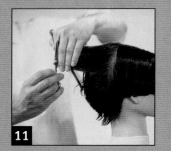

9. Using pivotal partings, bring sections from the back forward, toward the side guide, and cut. Work all the way to the center back.

10. In preparation for cutting the back, take a 1/2" (1.25 cm) vertical section from the center of the back. Hold it straight out from the curve of the head, and cut it vertically.

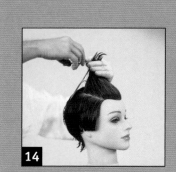

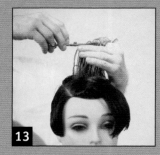

11. Bring the hair from both sides back to this stable guide and cut. Again, use 1/2" (1.25 cm) sections, and direct the hair back to your stable guide until you run out of length toward the ears.

12. Establish a guide for cutting the top front and crown areas. Part a horizontal section across the top of the head, positioned upward from the top of the ears.

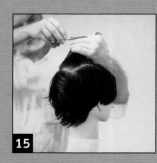

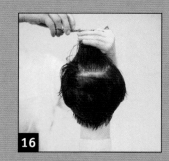

13. Comb and hold this section straight up, then cut it horizontally to establish your length guide.

14. Bring all the hair in front of this section back to the guide and cut.

15. Part upward from the top of the ear as a guide to begin sectioning into the crown area of the head. Bring the crown sections forward to the stable guide and cut.

16. Use 1/2" (1.25 cm) sections for control and cut until you no longer have enough length to reach the guide.

17. Part off the fringe to cut the front perimeter into the desired shape.

18. Use a pointing technique to create a softened edge.

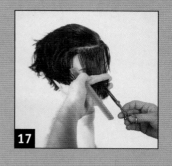
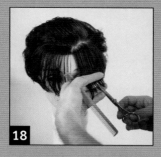

19. The layering technique used in this haircut has created weight corners.

20. These weight corners may be softened by holding the hair straight out from the curve of the head and pointing into the lengths to diffuse the edge.

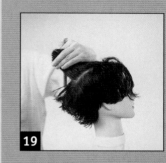
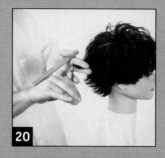

21. Use the pointing technique at the weight corner areas throughout the head.

22. Use the pointing technique in front of and over the ear, holding the hair with the comb.

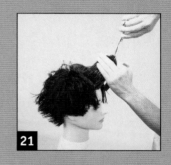
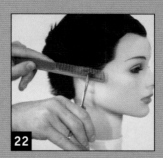

23. To complete the cut, refine the side edges. Strive for a soft, wispy effect, using variations on the pointing technique.

24. The finished style has dynamic movement and texture with a shape that allows for easily created volume and dimension.

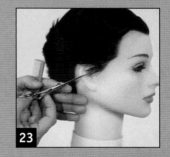
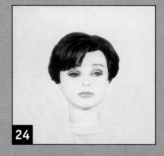

BLOW-DRYING LAYERED SQUARE SHAPE

OVERVIEW

The styling of shorter shapes is usually dictated by the way in which the hair was cut. Clients choose shorter shapes because they want ease of handling—so the finish should be easy care, too.

APPLY

With your clients, these technical steps will follow consultation, shampoo, and power or towel drying.

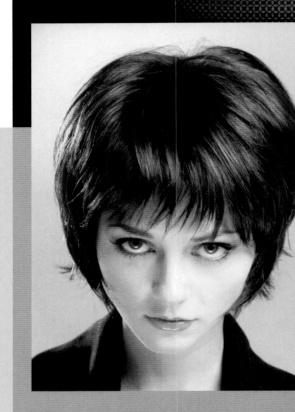

PROCEDURE

1. Distribute the hair into the style lines. Next, apply a styling product of your choice. Here a liquid gel is used for sleek control.

2. Work the product through the hair. A foam is applied to the crown area for more airy volume.

3. Begin to dry the front area. Direct the lengths and the air flow into the desired movement. The airflow is directed along the top surface. A vent brush facilitates even, thorough airflow.

4. Work around to the nape. Again the lengths are closely contoured.

5. Switch to a round brush and begin to work the crown area. The goal is to maximize volume in this area.

6. Continue through to the side section on either side, connecting with the directional placement in the crown.

7. Comb the hair with a wide-toothed texture comb.

8. Detail the ends with your fingers, using a small amount of spray or pomade on the fingertips.

9. Spray to finish. Lift for volume in the crown—balance the shape while spraying.

10. Use your creative artistry to finish this design. Directional movement, volume, and enhanced texture are all features of this finished style.

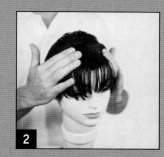
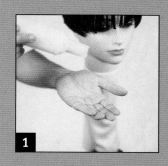
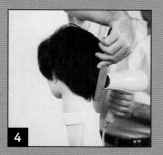
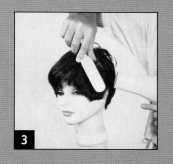
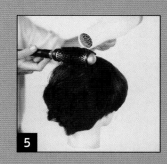
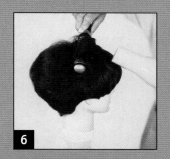
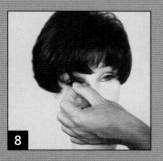
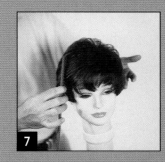
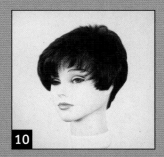
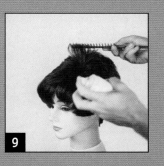

Getting an idea should be like sitting down on a pin; it should make you jump up and do something.

E.L. Simpson

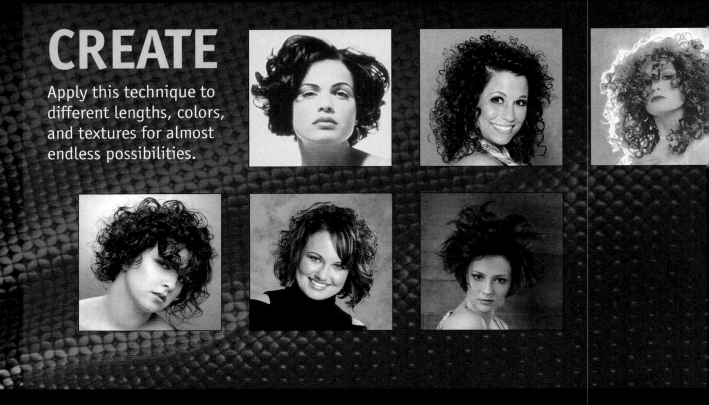

CREATE

Apply this technique to different lengths, colors, and textures for almost endless possibilities.

PERIMETER LAYERS

OVERVIEW

Long, layered shapes are an often-requested design in the salon. They are highly commercial and may be styled for a wide variety of looks. Soft, face-framing layers complement the long horizontal bluntness of the remainder of the cut.

To begin, you'll learn a fundamental approach to this cut. As you progress, you will start to introduce some of the many variations on this silhouette into your work.

APPLY

With your clients, these technical steps will follow the consultation and shampoo.

ON DVD ▶

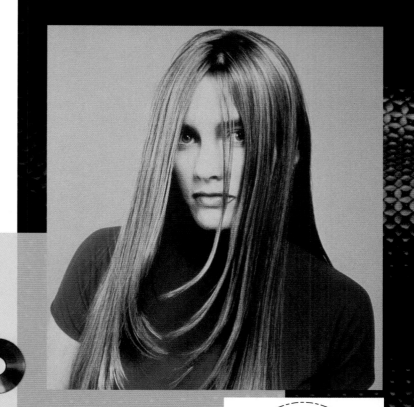

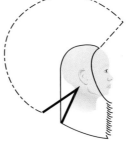

This shape features a horizontal blunt perimeter line combined with long, soft layers that flow from the jawline down to the blunt weight line.

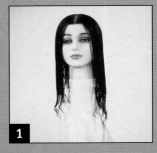

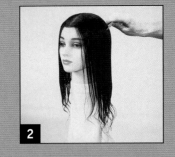

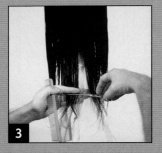

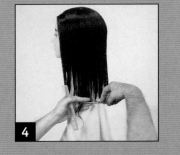

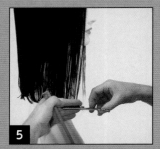

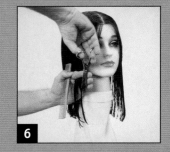

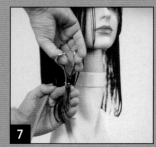

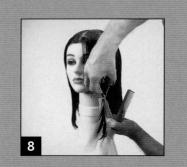

PROCEDURE

1. Comb the hair gently to remove any tangles. Create a center part.

2. Make certain the hair is evenly distributed all around the head in natural fall.

3. Begin removing excess length in the back, starting on the left back side. Use a horizontal cutting position; hold all the hair between your fingers and cut. You can also hold the hair flat with your comb and cut, using comb control alone.

4. Cut toward the side, using the horizontal cutting position with your palm downward. Complete this side.

5. Continue cutting horizontally toward the front right, following the same procedure. Make sure to maintain the natural fall position as you cut. Note the scissor position.

6. Part off a section that moves from the center part in front down to the sideburn area. Clip the remaining lengths out of the way. Hold this section of the hair downward between the first and middle finger of your hand at the jawline. Angle the fingers diagonally, with the tips of the fingers pointing toward the chin.

7. With your other hand, hold your scissors against the hand with the hair and begin to slide both hands down in unison as you open and close the blades along the hair to remove length. Continue moving steadily downward, making certain you maintain natural fall. Stop when you reach the bottom weight line, where you run out of hair.

8. Cut the opposite side in the same manner, layering the hair by sliding your scissors down the entire front perimeter as you open and close the blades. Note the holding, cutting, and scissor positions being used.

9. Cross-check the two sides for evenness, parting off a small, horizontal section at the front, combing it down, and making sure the two sides meet at the same point and blend.

10. Option: To create a looser, more highly textured effect, take the same partings as before, but comb and elevate the hair forward. Cut the hair diagonally, slide cutting as before. More layers will result.

11. This shape is highly desirable for many clients. The possible variations with this slide-cutting technique allow for the creation of a multitude of effects.

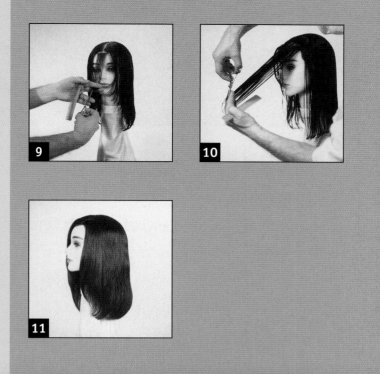

Success is a journey, not a destination. The doing is usually more important than the outcome.

Arthur Ashe

CREATE

Apply this technique to different lengths, colors, and textures for almost endless possibilities.

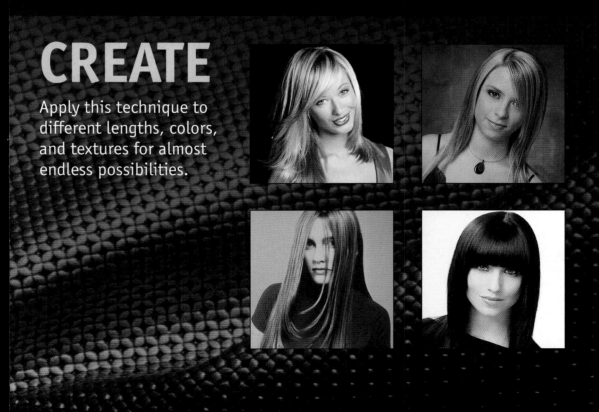

LIGHT LAYERS

OVERVIEW

This shape is a true classic—and yet very contemporary as well! Internal layers flow over the perimeter blunt cut. The longer layers in this cut are preplanned according to the initial guideline that you create around the front hairline; you'll bring all internal layers to this length. The use of this stable guide will make for shorter layers around the front hairline, increasing to longer layers at the crown and back of the head.

APPLY

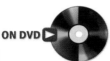

With your clients, these technical steps will follow the consultation and shampoo.

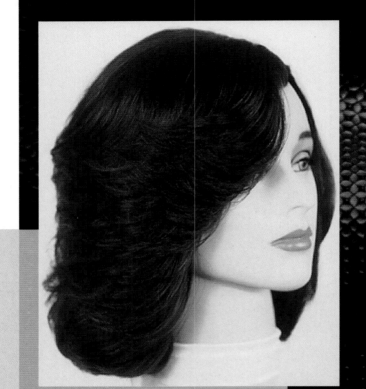

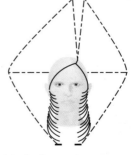

This haircut features long or "light" layers that flow over the perimeter blunt haircut. More layers frame the front area and move toward a lesser amount at the center back of the head.

PROCEDURE

1. Comb the hair in natural fall and establish a side part on the left side. Create a blunt cut, following the steps for the horizontal blunt.

2. Locate the natural fringe area by parting a triangular section from the side part to the recession area, at the outside corner of the eye. Part off a 1/2" (1.25 cm) horizontal section from the front and clip the remainder of the section out of the way. Use a point of reference on the face, such as the lip, for where you'll begin cutting diagonally back.

3. Direct the hair in natural fall and position your fingers diagonally; position the scissors to follow the same diagonal line your fingers form. Begin cutting near the lip and follow the angle of your fingers. Cut the entire fringe section to this guide.

4. Repeat this procedure on the opposite side of the part. Pick up the hair at the recession area of the right side. Cut diagonally from the lip line back, just as you did before.

5. Section out a rectangle section through the interior of the head.

6. Begin at the front hairline area by taking a horizontal parting from the front of the section.

7. Hold this section straight up from the top of the head and begin cutting out diagonally about 6 inches from the scalp. This will be your stable guide.

8. Hold the stable guide straight up from the top of the head and bring partings to it as you cut on a slightly upward angle from the side part outward. Work from the front to the back of the section, taking partings and directing them to the initial stable guide until you complete the section. This technique will create a length increase.

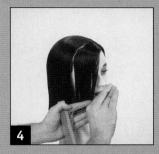

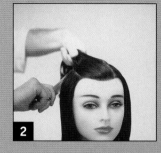

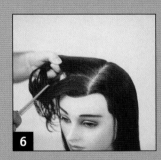

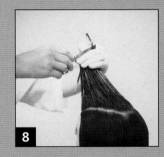

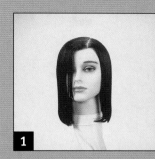

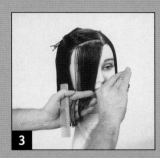

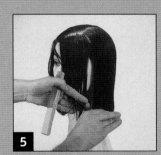

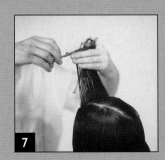

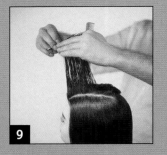

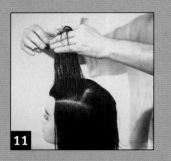

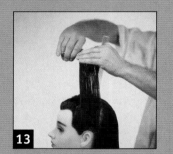

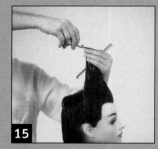

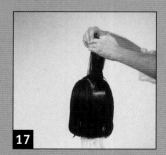

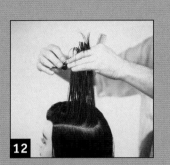

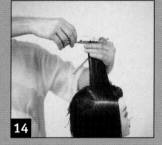

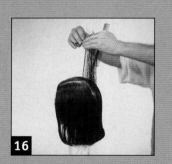

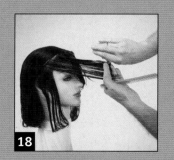

9. Cross-check these internal lengths by taking a vertical parting from the front to the crown. Note how the angle moves from shorter at the front . . .

10. . . . to longer at the crown area. Direct lengths straight up and check the line.

11. Use this internal length increase as your guideline for cutting the sides. Part vertically through the side. Using a section of hair from the top as the guideline, bring sections straight up, distributing the hair neatly to the stable guide, then cut to this guide along the diagonal line created.

12. Moving back, bring lengths straight up to the stable guide for cutting. Notice how the fingers of the holding hand are angled diagonally upward from front to back.

13. Continue layering one side until you run out of hair. This will be where you meet the lengths from the horizontal blunt.

14. Move to the opposite side and begin bringing sections to the stable guides and cutting diagonally.

15. Continue layering that side until completed.

16. Blend the crown lengths into the top area. Use pivotal partings to work around the back crown area. Direct lengths straight up from the top of the head and begin cutting out diagonally using the predetermined length/guide from the top.

17. Continue this procedure through the crown to complete the layering.

18. After completing the layering, check the cut response. Finish the cut by checking the line framing the face. Direct lengths forward and position the fingers outward from the fringe length cut earlier to refine the line.

19. Repeat the procedure on the other side.

20. The finished silhouette shows the long layers that have been created. These layers will allow for movement, surface texture, and dimension to be achieved in the finished style. The cut is very versatile and can be styled in a variety of ways, whether back from the face or forward onto the face.

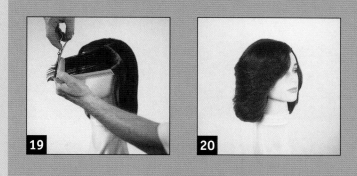

If you can imagine it, you can achieve it. If you can dream it, you can become it.

William Arthur Ward

CREATE

Apply this technique to different lengths, colors, and textures for almost endless possibilities.

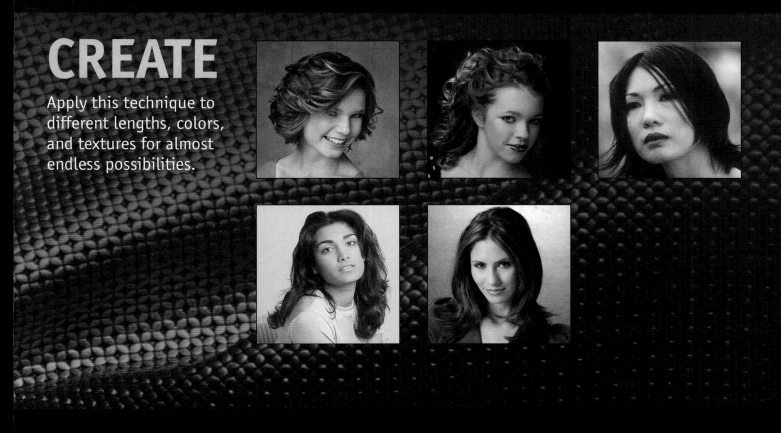

OVERVIEW

This shape's heavily layered or textured effect comes from the cutting technique used throughout the interior. It can be worn straight or in a full, voluminous look; it can be styled forward or back. It provides the client with great versatility.

APPLY

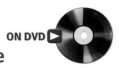 ON DVD ▶

With your clients, these technical steps will follow the consultation and shampoo.

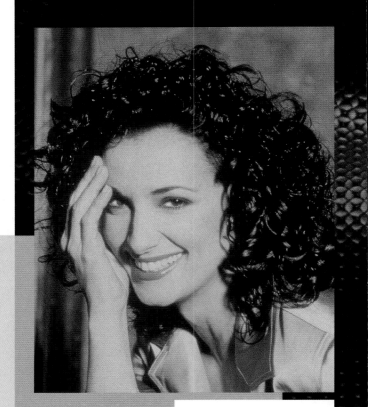

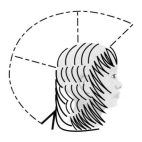

In this heavily layered shape, lengths progress from short layers through the interior to longer layers at the exterior. The layers provide textured volume.

PROCEDURE

1. On a client you may first need to establish the perimeter length and shape. Create a diagonal back blunt style off a center part. Create a center part and take a 1/2" (1.25 cm) section along the top front hairline.

2. Comb and hold the hair downward over the face at low elevation. Use a point of reference on the face, such as the lip, to establish the length, cutting horizontally.

3. Section through the entire side hairline area. Direct and hold the hair with your fingers positioned diagonally. Cut the side lengths to blend from the fringe to the exterior length. Repeat on the other side, cutting diagonally.

4. Part out a rectangular section through the top from the front hairline to the crown.

5. Part out a horizontal section at the front hairline. Hold the previously established front guide straight up from the top of the head.

6. Cut horizontally.

7. Use this section as a traveling guide. Pick up a small portion of it with each newly parted section and cut horizontally, moving back toward the crown. Continue to use the same holding position (straight up from the top of the head) and horizontal cutting position throughout.

8. Cross-check your work through this top area by taking vertical sections and holding them straight up from the top of the head. Clean up any unevenness.

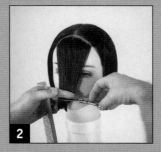
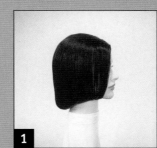

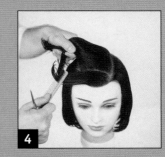
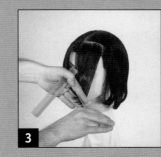

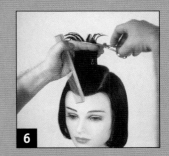
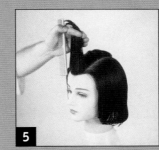

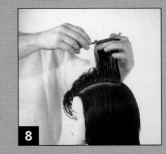
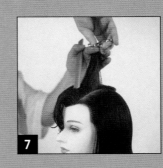

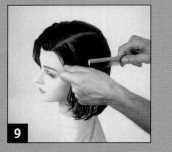

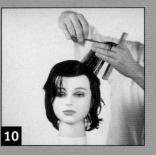

9. Section through the crest area. Part off a vertical section at the front hairline. Direct this section up and out from the crest area.

10. Begin cutting out with your fingers in the position shown. This connects to the length from the top.

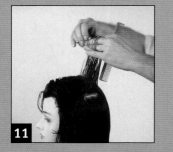

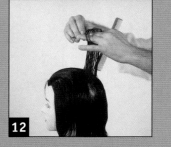

11. Use the first section as a traveling guide to cut the sections behind it. Angle the fingers diagonally and continue cutting out.

12. Take radial partings from the crown as you move from the side toward the center back, cutting out to the established guide line.

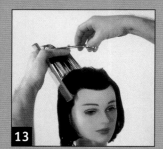

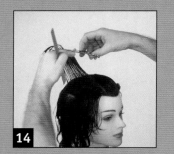

13., 14. Repeat the steps on the right side, starting with the establishment of the traveling guide.

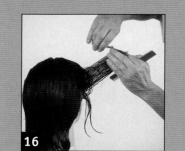

15. Work back and use radial partings as you move around the crown. Continue until you reach the center back.

16. In this technique you are cutting toward the perimeter. Continue this technique to the center back as a control measure for blending all lengths outward.

OVERVIEW

This technique for drying textured or overcurly hair will distort the curl as little as possible, giving the hair a clean and healthy look that's free from frizziness. You'll use both a vent brush and a blow-dryer, allowing you to lift the hair for quick drying and natural separation.

APPLY

With your clients, these technical steps will follow consultation, shampoo, and power or towel drying.

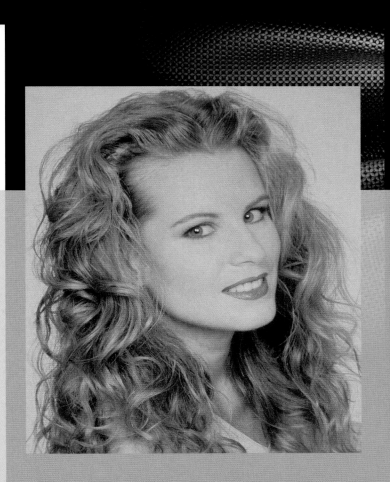

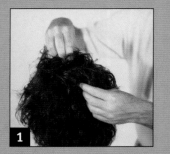

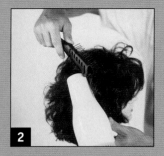

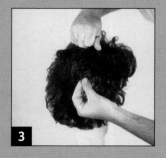

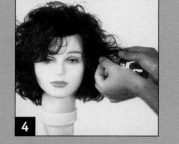

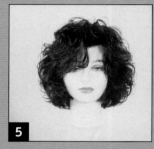

PROCEDURE

1. Thoroughly towel dry the hair. Apply a styling product of your choice and work it through the hair.

2. Use a vent brush to provide thorough, effective air flow onto the hair while creating volume.

3. Use small, gentle finger movements to separate the hair.

4. Finish the design by separating the textured hair with the tips of your fingers.

5. The finished style shows enhanced textural movement and volume.

CREATE

Apply this technique to different lengths, colors, and textures for almost endless possibilities.

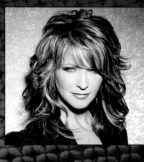
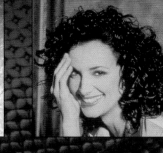
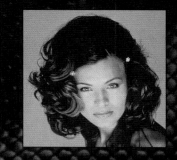

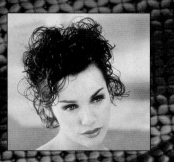
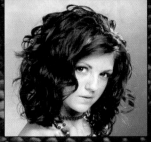
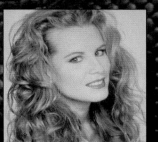
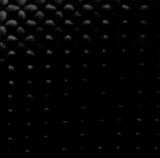

HEAVY LAYERS ON PRESSED HAIR

OVERVIEW

A client who prefers to wear her curly hair in a smooth and straight finished style has two choices: Either chemically relax the hair or press the natural curl into a smooth texture. If the client chooses the nonchemical pressing alternative, you must first press the hair smooth and then cut it dry. This will ensure the creation of the most accurate, precise shape.

Techniques for straightening hair have come and gone through the years, but applying heat to dry curly hair along with pressure is a method that has endured. Pressing hair to straighten it will always be a popular technique, and it's important to know the proper method for cutting a pressed head of hair.

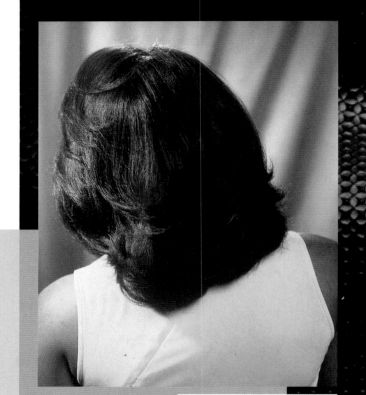

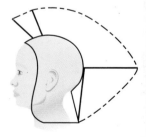

Heavy layers flow through the interior and along the perimeter frame that has been cut blunt.

While many haircuts are performed on damp hair, hair that has been pressed will be cut dry. Not only does the dry method maintain the straightening achieved by pressing, but it also permits greater precision in creating the shape because you can perfectly predict where the hair will fall in the finished style. Whether dried straight and smooth or dried naturally, a precise shape is ensured.

APPLY

ON DVD ▷

Before beginning this service, blow-dry the hair and press with a pressing iron. After you complete the cut, curl the hair to add soft movement and body.

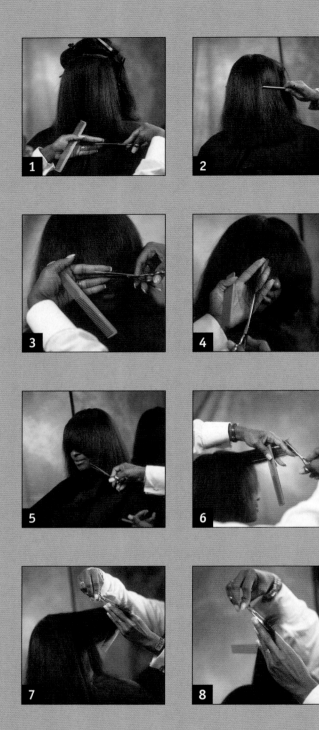

PROCEDURE

1. Divide the hair into four sections: crown area, right side, left side, and back. Starting at the center back, hold the hair straight down and cut a horizontal line using a low (one-finger) elevation. Work toward the left side.

2. Release the hair in the crown area. Notice that the previously cut layers do not reach the blunt perimeter. These lengths will get cut during the layering process. Move to the right side of the back section, comb the hair down, and cut.

3. At the front of the head, comb the fringe section forward and, using the tip of the nose as a guide, cut straight across and adjacent to the outside corner of the eye. Repeat to cut the other half of the fringe.

4. Move to the side of the head. Comb the side and top sections slightly forward and, using the front fringe area as a guide, cut the side at a diagonal from the nose down, blending it with the fringe area framing the face.

5. Move to the other side and continue framing the face, blending the hair at a diagonal with the fringe area.

6. Move to the top front area. Make partings so that they pivot around the crown. Part out a pie-shaped section from the top center crown to the front hairline. Hold the hair straight out from the front of the head and begin cutting out along the fingers to create a length increase.

7. Move around the head, continuing to part out sections that radiate from the crown, holding them straight out from the side of the head and cutting out to the traveling guide that you've created.

8. Move through the crown of the head. Hold the hair straight out from the curve of the head and begin cutting out.

9. The haircut was curled to complete the style. The completed style has fluid movement and frames the face with a soft fringe.

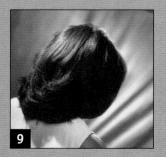

OVERVIEW

A press and curl is a temporary thermal straightening technique used for very curly hair; the hair will revert to its natural state when shampooed. It may also be affected by perspiration, humidity, or other elements. No chemicals are used in this service—some clients do not want chemicals in their hair. If they are on medication, pregnant, or have extremely dry scalps, clients will want a press and curl because it is chemical-free.

APPLY

With your clients, these technical steps will follow consultation, shampoo, and power or towel drying.

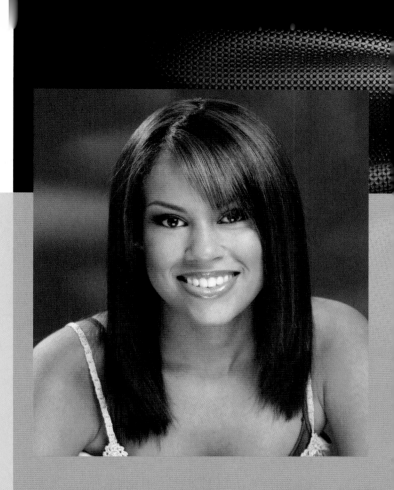

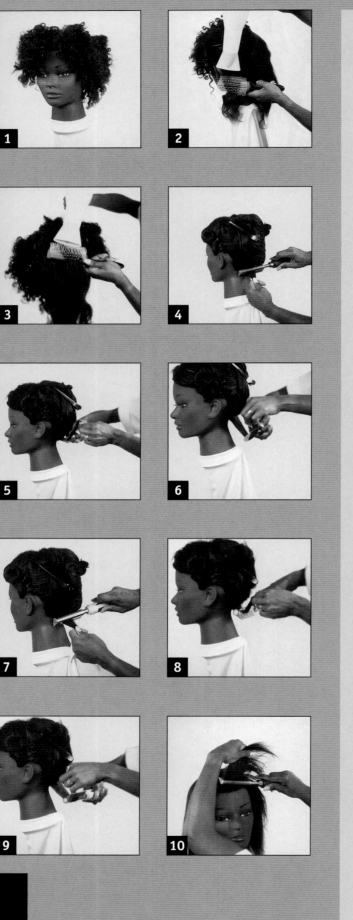

PROCEDURE

1. Shampooing the hair before a press and curl is not recommended when working on a mannequin. Working with dry hair allows you greater manageability.

2. Divide the head into four quadrants. Work your way up through the first section of hair using a blow-dryer with nozzle and a hard rubber brush to heat and straighten the hair. Work section by section, then stretch through the top surface.

3. Continue this technique through all sections of the head to prepare for the pressing.

4. Divide the hair into four quadrants. Divide each section into 1 1/2" (3.75 cm) horizontal sections. Both an electric pressing comb and a thermal comb should be tested before being placed on the hair. Holding the hair firmly in one hand and your pressing comb in the other, direct the teeth of the pressing comb into the hair as close to the scalp as possible. Comb outward to the ends. Turn the back of the pressing comb to press the section.

5. Press the comb through the hair, rotating it to bring the barrel against the lengths. The teeth guide the hair only; the barrel does the straightening. As you finish each rotation, the teeth of the comb should be pointing toward you.

6. Hold the hair as you move down the shaft until you've pressed the very end of the hair. Keep the hair taut to facilitate straightening.

7. You would use the same technique with an electric pressing comb.

8. Note how the pressing comb is turned while working down the length of the hair.

9. While the technique of pressing with an electric comb is the same as with a thermal comb, you will have to go over the hair two to three times more.

10. When you've finished the interior, press the hair along the perimeter. Hold the hair with a gentle but firm tension as you pull the comb through the hair.

11. No sectioning is needed when you press the hair along the perimeter.

12. Holding the hair firmly, continue pressing the outer perimeter hairline.

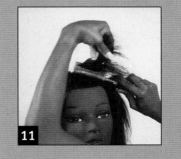
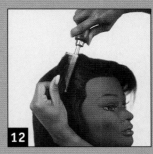

13. Divide the hair into four sections starting at the nape. Test the heat of the iron by placing it on a white paper towel. Take up one of these 1 1/2" (3.75 cm) sections and test your curling iron by placing it on top of the section. Slide the iron down the hair shaft while firmly holding the hair—this is called silking the hair. Remember to always leave the curling iron slightly open until you get to the end of the hair.

14. Hold the hair and slightly open curling iron. Firmly slide the curling iron down the hair.

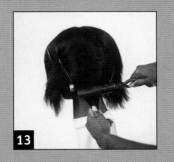
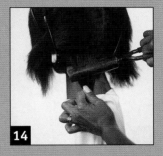

15. When you get to the ends of the hair, close the curling iron and work the ends of the hair into the middle of the curl.

16. Placing a hard rubber comb under the curling iron is imperative if you are going to roll the curling iron to the scalp.

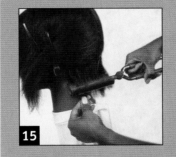
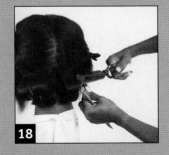

17. Hold the curling iron in the hair until you can no longer see the ends of the hair. Slide the iron out of the curl.

18. Slide the curling iron until you reach the end of the hair.

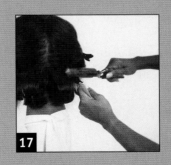
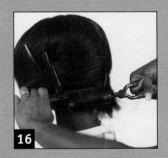

19. Use a hard rubber comb to protect the scalp.

20. Place the styling comb between the scalp and curling iron to protect the scalp. Work upward toward the crown.

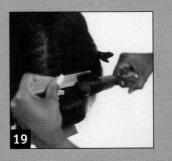
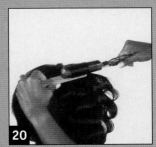

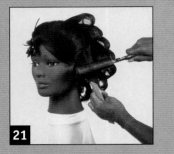 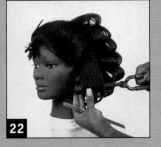

21. Moving to the side, continue curling the hair.

22. When you are not rolling the curling iron toward the scalp, be sure to direct it away from the client's scalp with your hand. Place your fingers between the client's face and the curling iron.

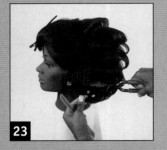 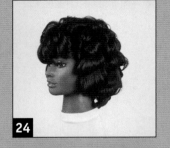

23. Complete the curling technique by moving up the section of hair into the interior.

24. The press and curl is complete and ready to be styled. Notice the smooth lines of the curls.

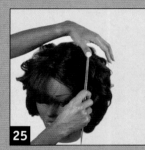 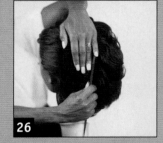

25. Using a rake-type styling comb, comb the hair toward the back of the head.

26. As the rake-type styling comb moves toward the back center of the head, smooth your hand over the hair in the same direction.

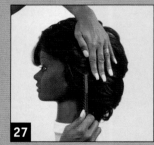 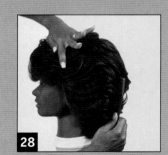

27. As you reach the center back of the head, stop and, applying pressure, push the hair toward the front.

28. Pushing the hair toward the front will create a layered look.

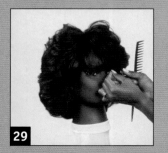 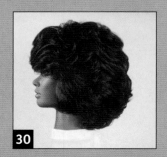

29. Repeat on other side, pulling out pieces of hair to softly frame the face. Detail the surface for the desired textural movement.

30. The styled press and curl creates a softened shape with textural and directional movement and dimension.

Cherish your visions and your dreams as they are the children of your soul; the blueprints of your ultimate achievements.

Napoleon Hill

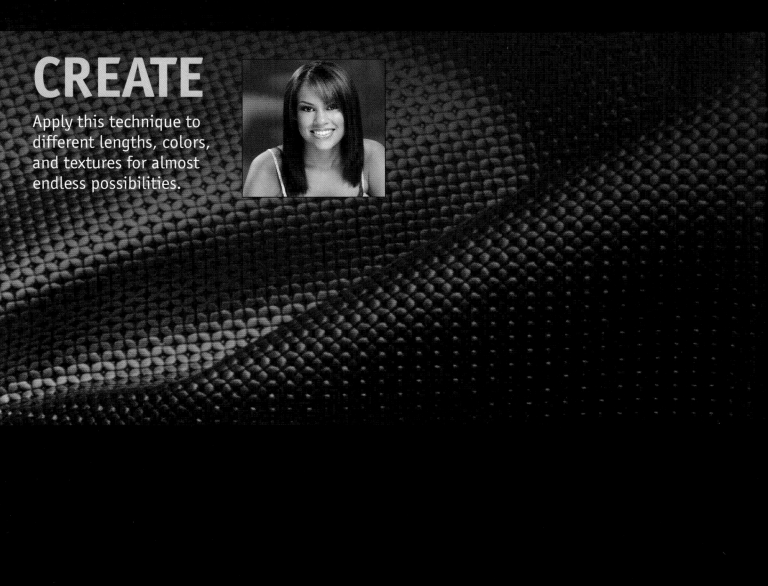

CREATE

Apply this technique to different lengths, colors, and textures for almost endless possibilities.

FULL LAYERS

OVERVIEW

In this shape, the entire haircut is progressively layered—shorter lengths in the interior work toward longer lengths around the perimeter. This silhouette has been called a shag or a shake, as well as simply being defined as a full head of overall layers with longer lengths around the perimeter.

APPLY

ON DVD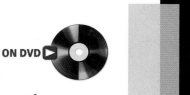

With your clients, these technical steps will follow the consultation and shampoo.

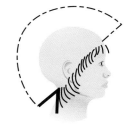

Shown here is the completely layered shape. Lengths move progressively from short layers in the interior to long on the exterior.

PROCEDURE

1. Comb the hair in natural fall. Part out a rectangular section from the front hairline to the crown and upward from the center of the eye on either side.

2. Part a 1/2" (1.25 cm) section from the front of the section at the hairline. Comb and hold at a low elevation and cut it horizontally to the tip of the nose.

3. Holding the hair in natural fall, connect and blend this fringe length diagonally through the sides.

4. Release horizontal sections through the interior. Use the initially cut section to establish the traveling guide. Each section is held straight out from the curve of the head and cut horizontally.

5. Work all the way back to the crown, picking up a portion of the previously cut section each time to act as a traveling guide. Comb and distribute the hair neatly out from the head and cut horizontally.

6. Having completed the top area, part out vertical sections through the crest area for layering through this panel. Direct the lengths straight up and out from the head and begin cutting out toward the perimeter area using a traveling guide.

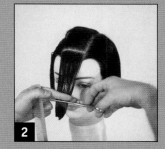

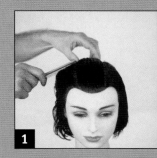

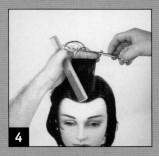

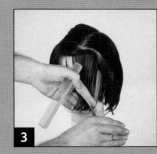

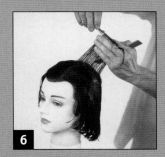

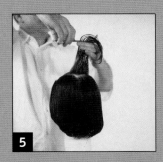

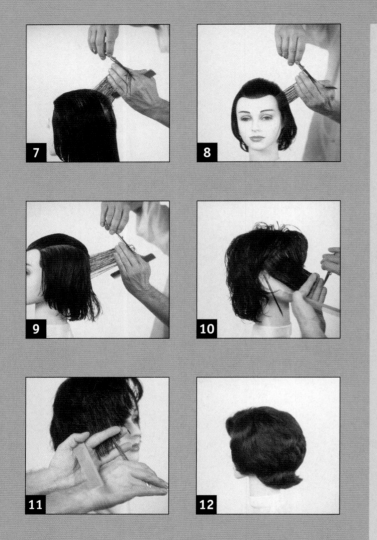

7. Continue this holding and cutting position to the center back. The partings radiate around the crown area.

8. Move to the next panel. Part off vertically, holding the hair straight, and begin cutting out to blend to the perimeter frame.

9. Using this section as a traveling guide, work toward the center back, cutting the side panels. The panels should be about 2" (5 cm) wide. Check through the nape lengths with vertical sections. Cross-check your work by pulling sections out horizontally. Work through the entire haircut in this manner.

10. To complete the cut, check and refine the entire perimeter frame area.

11. Detail the front perimeter to suit the face. Here, point cutting softens the look. Place the fingers according to the depth of pointing that will be made into the ends of the hair. Observe and check the softness as it's developing.

12. The layered cut gives the hair a lot of movement. The finished style shows the cut with a subtle flip in the nape area. This shape offers a multitude of styling options.

Wealth is not his that has it, but his that enjoys it.

Benjamin Franklin

OVERVIEW

Here's another example of styling the hair to conform to the contours of its shape. The finished style highlights the shape of the cut, and the drying technique you use accentuates the layering above the ears and through the top of the head.

APPLY

With your clients, these technical steps will follow consultation, shampoo, and power or towel drying.

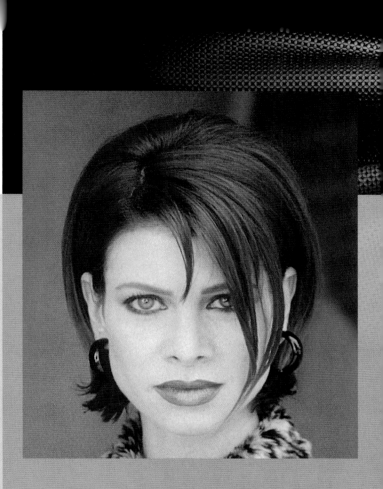

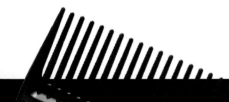

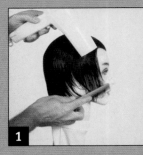

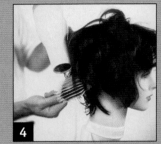

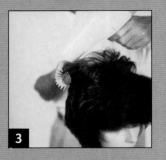

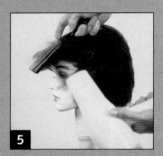

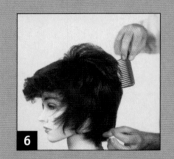

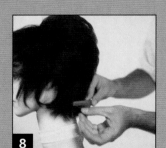

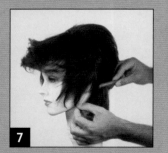

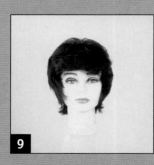

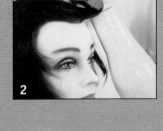

PROCEDURE

1. Apply a styling product of your choice and work it through the hair. Holding the hair very close around the perimeter shape with a comb, dry the hair, following the comb with the dryer. This will keep this area very closely contoured.

2. Move to the fringe area next. Using a rubber-based blow-drying brush, overdirect the hair to create volume and fullness. Note how flat the base area is held when turning the ends back and toward the side.

3. Continue into the crown area.

4. Comb through the nape area if it needs lift.

5. Blend and connect the side sections with the front.

6. Use a texture comb to separate and detail the lengths. Back comb the crown area, then detail, using your comb and fingers.

7. Continue detailing. This is where your artistry is expressed.

8. Detail the edges. Spray for the desired hold.

9. The finished style shows closely contoured layers through the exterior with an emphasis on directional volume through the fringe and crown areas.

The difference between the impossible and the possible lies in a person's determination.

Tommy Lasorda

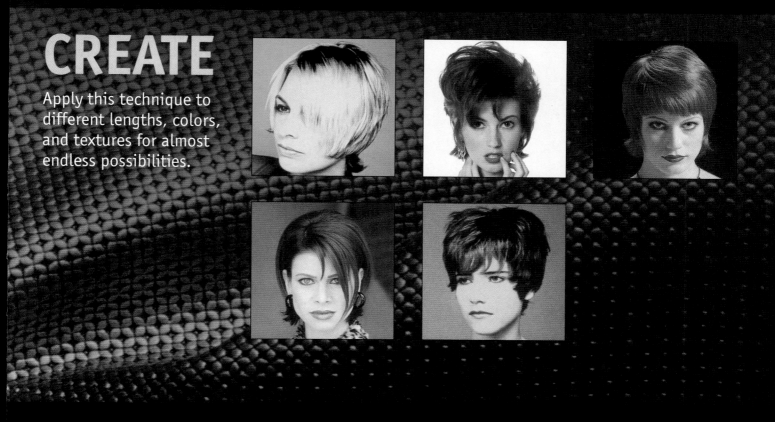

CREATE

Apply this technique to different lengths, colors, and textures for almost endless possibilities.

LAYERED GRADUATION WITH CLIPPERS

OVERVIEW

Clipper cutting decreases cutting time—which means faster service. Using this free-form method will give you very accurate results because it offers precision in creating lines. Generally, when you use a clipper, the emphasis of the cut will be on the silhouette. For extra control, some stylists use both hands to hold the clipper. If you're holding the clipper with one hand and the hair or a comb with your other, remember that the more tension you use, the more precise the line your clipper will create. Before you begin any cut with your clipper, however, you must envision where you are going with it.

APPLY

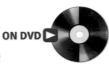

With your clients, these technical steps will follow the consultation and pressing.

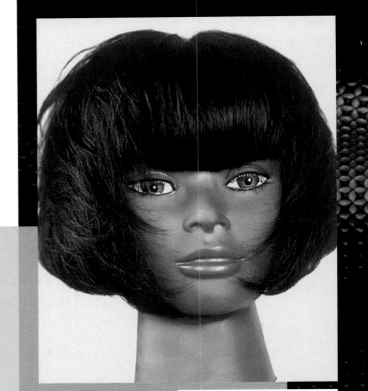

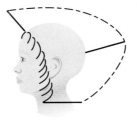

In this design, interior layers flow over the perimeter graduation. A blunt fringe adds dramatic flair. Precise lines are easily created using the clipper cutting technique.

PROCEDURE

1. Before beginning, examine the clipper blade to ensure that it is in top-notch condition. Clean and oil the clipper regularly. Begin by doing a rough cut through the back area to remove excess length. Work methodically with the blade inverted against the hair as shown.

2. Establish the perimeter frame through the back of the head. Point the clipper blade toward the neck and use the clipper to create the line from ear to ear.

3. At the front of the head, section off the fringe area. For instructional purposes only, a piece of white cardboard has been clipped under the fringe. Cut first at the center of the forehead area, then extend the line outward on either side to the outside corners of the eyes. Leave the fringe slightly longer if you intend to use an iron, which will make the fringe look shorter.

4. Move to the left side. Establish a new length for the side. This design length does not connect to the back section. From the tip of the earlobe to the jawline is the ideal length on the appropriate head shape.

5. Note the new position used here to sweep the blade sideways along the line. Cut to refine.

6. Create the same perimeter line on the other side. This freehand inverted clipper position works well when cutting a line against the skin. If cutting away from the head, hold the hair between the fingers.

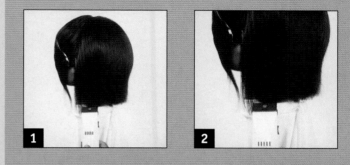
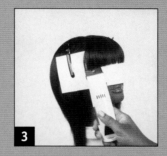
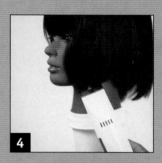
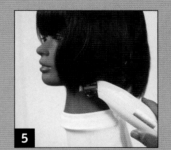
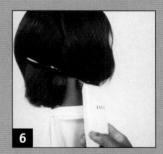

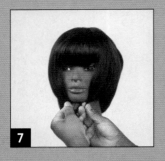

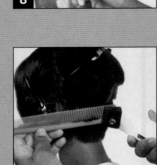

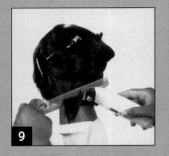

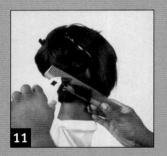

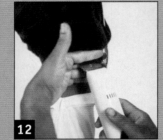

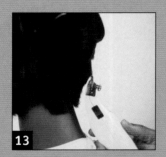

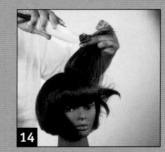

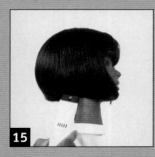

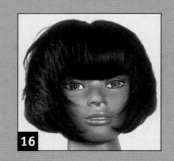

7. Using your mirror and standing directly in front of the head, check for balance in the length of your cut.

8. Using a clipper-over-comb technique, taper the neckline area. Hold a section of hair straight out from the curve of the head with the comb angled as shown. Establish your first cut with the clipper. Remember to envision where you are going with the cut.

9. Continue to create graduation toward the outer edges of the nape, using the clipper-over-comb technique. As you work toward the occipital bone, allow your elevation to move gradually outward from the neckline.

10. The comb here is slightly beveled—closer to the head along the back edge of the comb and farther away from the head along its teeth. Note the high graduation developing through this area.

11. Consistency in angling the comb, hair length, and graduation is essential. Blend from the center area toward the area behind the ear.

12. When you're cutting to blend the remainder of the back to the graduated nape area, control the hair lengths for cutting between the fingers.

13. Refine the sculptured shape for softness and precision using the clipper.

14. Through the top of the head, you will use a condensed cutting technique with large sections that radiate around the curve of the head. Comb a large section up behind the fringe. Begin cutting out from the fringe to the crown lengths. You will use this as a guide to move around the head with radial sections cutting out.

15. Comb and check the cut around the entire perimeter of the head for detail, trimming any uneven hair.

16. The finished style is smooth and voluminous, with graduation creating body at the nape.

OVERVIEW

Wrapping is a technique for keeping straightened hair smooth. The hair design can be left as is, close to the head, or combed out. You can also create wrapped styles with extra volume by using rollers that are wrapped in a single direction at the top. This traditional wrap technique will create a style that lasts as long as a week. It's perfect for active clients—it makes hair more manageable and gives it added movement. This can be done on wet or dry hair.

APPLY

With your clients, these technical steps will follow consultation, shampoo, and power or towel drying. The finished style is created through the use of a wrapping technique. This creates a smooth, glossy texture.

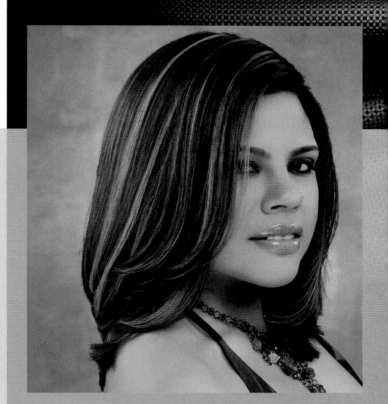

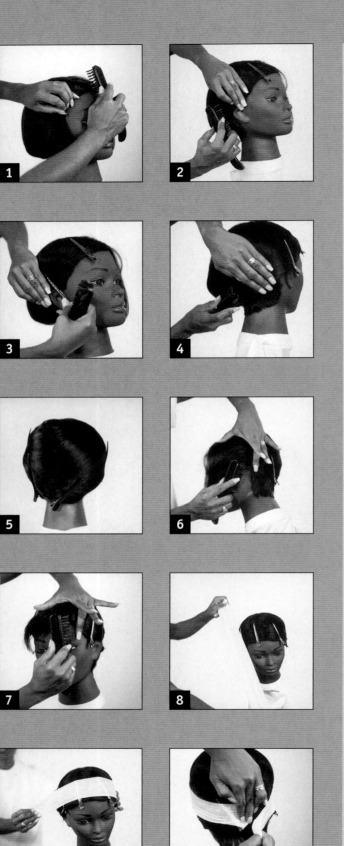

PROCEDURE

1. Brush the hair around the outer perimeter of the head.

2. Holding the hair in place with long clips, continue brushing around the outer perimeter of the head until you reach your starting point.

3. As your hands move, your body should also move in sync around your client's head.

4. Make sure you keep the hair low so it remains on the outer perimeter of the head.

5. At this stage in the wrapping process, you can see how the hair smoothly follows the contour of the head.

6. Continue bringing the hair around the head, holding your hand securely. (A pivotal movement is used.)

7. As you brush, continue placing long clips. Brush up and around toward the top front of the head, clipping as you go.

8. Stretch a neck strip around the entire head.

9. Place the neck strip over the clips.

10. Stretch the neck strip so it overlaps at the ends.

11. Holding the neck strip in place, start removing the clips. Remove the back clip first because you will need this area free for securing the ends of the neck strip.

12. Secure the wrapped strip with a bobby pin.

13., 14. Start removing the rest of the clips from the head.

15. If you have been working on a dry head, you will need to leave the hair wrapped for about 15 minutes. If the hair was wet, you will need to place the client under a dryer for 45 minutes to 1 hour, depending on the hair length, until the hair is completely dry. The longer you leave the hair wrapped, the smoother it will be.

16. Unwrap the hair and brush the straightened hair into the desired style. Shown here is one possible comb out of the wrapped hair.

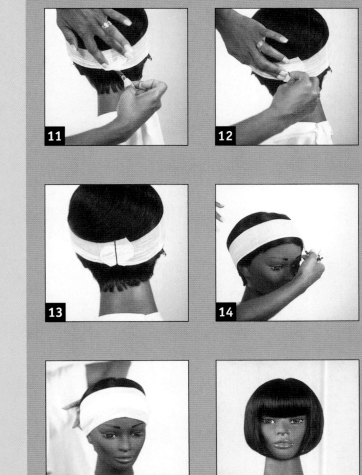

CREATE

pply this technique to ifferent lengths, colors, nd textures for almost ndless possibilities.

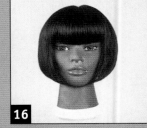

HIGH GRADUATION

OVERVIEW

In this style, you will create high graduation throughout the entire back area of the cut to blend and harmonize with the layered shape that frames the face through the top and sides. This cut defines the head shape through the back area by the closer contours of the graduation; the layered lengths around the face frame it attractively, adding a soft, feminine touch as well as versatility.

APPLY

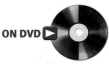
ON DVD ▶

With your clients, these technical steps will follow the consultation and shampoo.

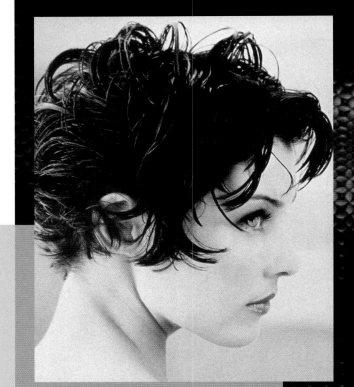

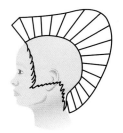

This versatile shape combines a high graduation through the back with soft layers that frame the face.

PROCEDURE

1. Comb the hair in natural fall. Create a side part. Distribute the hair around the curve of the head in natural fall.

2. Move to the back and part out a 1/2" (1.25 cm) section from crown to nape.

3. Starting at the top of the section, hold the hair straight back from the crown area, angling the fingers outward from the curve of the head. Begin cutting in along the section, angling toward the nape.

4. Continue down the section, cutting in closer to the head as you approach the nape. This will be your traveling guide for the top and sides. Notice the holding position, straight out from the curve of the head, as you work from the crest area down.

5. Finish cutting the traveling guide at the nape, directly below the section you just cut.

6. Part out the next vertical section and cut along the traveling guide, using the same holding position and cutting angle. Continue parting and cutting vertical sections. Take a small portion of the first section you cut, hold it with the next vertical section, and move from the back toward the sides, cutting sections to the same angle as the traveling guide. Let the guide travel slightly toward the new section being cut.

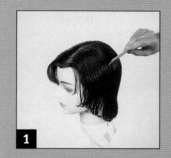

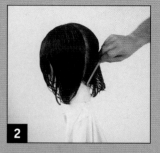

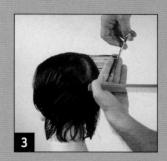

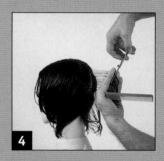

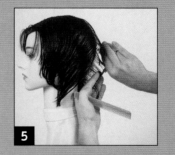

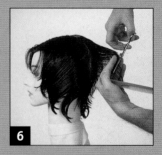

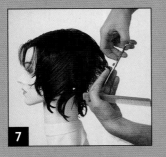

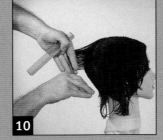

7. Part out vertically, pivoting around the crown. Follow the traveling guide forward, cutting from the top section toward the nape. Always pull the hair straight out from the curve of the head and use the cutting-in position along the guide.

8. Continue cutting the back and sides until you reach the ear area.

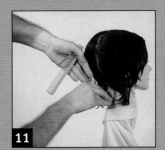

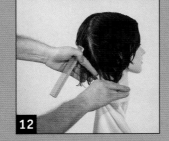

9. The last back section that you cut, which is behind the ear, will now serve as a stable guide to which you will bring all the side lengths. Hold the section above the ear straight out from the curve of the head. Direct all side lengths back to this guide, section by section, and use the cutting in position along the pre-established line. This will create the layered effect through the front.

10. Move to the opposite side. Pick up your traveling guide to follow.

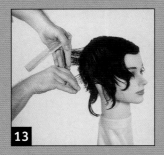

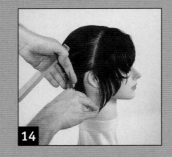

11. Complete each vertical section, using the same technique that you used on the left side.

12. The vertical sections that you are cutting radiate around the head. Make sure you follow your traveling guide, which should be visible at all times.

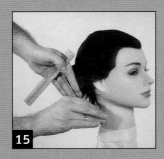

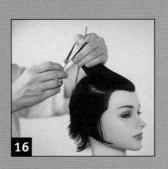

13. Stop using a traveling guide when you reach the ear area, as you did on the left side.

14. At this point, you'll switch to a stable guide, as you did before. Bring sections back to this guide.

15. Continue using the stable guide to cut the remainder of the side, bringing 1/2" (1.25 cm) sections back to it.

16. Bring top sections back to the crown to check and blend internal lengths across the top of the head. Cross-check throughout the cut, cleaning up any unevenness.

17. In the finished cut, graduated effects make for much textural movement.

18. Refine the perimeter of the cut, working with the facial shape and hair texture. A slicing technique is used here to soften and variegate the perimeter line.

19. The finished shape has a diffused softness to it. The face-framing layers blend harmoniously with the graduated back area. This is a versatile and very desirable shape to suit a multitude of clients.

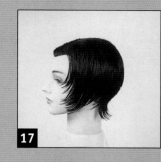

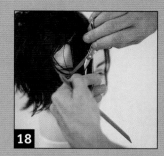

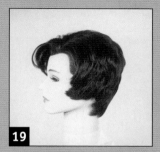

BLOW-DRYING HIGH GRADUATION

OVERVIEW

This style begins with the high graduation cut you completed in the haircutting part of this program. As with many shorter styles, you should use tools in the drying process to conform to the shape of the cut. The key to finishing this style is moving the brush through the hair as you direct heat from the dryer onto it.

APPLY

With your clients, these technical steps will follow consultation, shampoo, and power or towel drying.

In this design, the highly graduated haircut has been styled for a backswept flow away from the face.

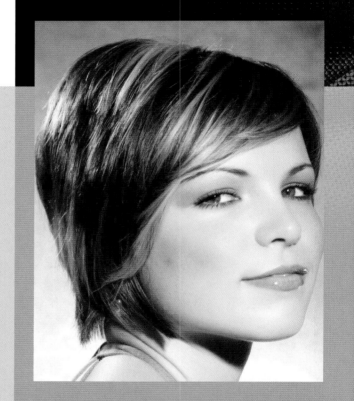

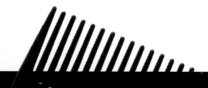

PROCEDURE

1. Apply a styling product of your choice and work it through the hair. Comb and direct the hair into the style lines in preparation for blow-drying.

2. Use a metal vent brush to wave a C-shaped section while following the brush with your dryer. Insert the brush into the hair and form a curved movement. Direct the air flow into the movement. Repeat on the opposite side.

3. Follow through to the ends of the hair. The brush is used to mold movement. Follow the brush with the blow-dryer, tracing in a curvature movement.

4. Use a round brush to lift and bend the hair around the face in a directional manner. Use this technique throughout the sides. Brush the hair in back to contour and blend to surrounding lengths. Use a spray, texture creme, or silicone shiner for the desired finish.

5. The finished style enhances the graduated movement through the back and the layers that frame the face.

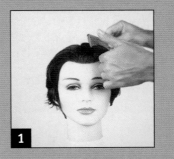
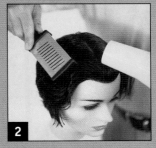
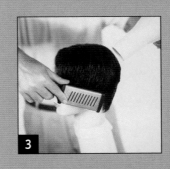
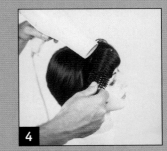
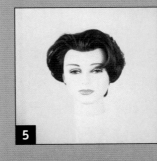
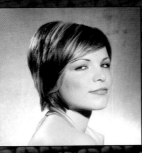
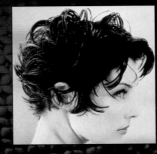
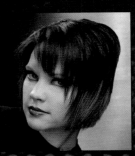
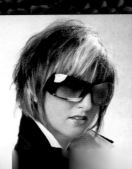
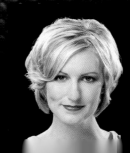

CREATE

pply this technique to ifferent lengths, colors, nd textures for almost ndless possibilities.

Destiny is not a matter of chance, it is a matter of choice. It is not a thing to be waited for, it is a thing to be achieved.

William Jennings Bryan

LAYERED RAZOR CUT

OVERVIEW

The razor is a superb tool for making the hair fluid and supple. Razor cutting tapers the lengths, creating a variety of lengths, and eliminates any angularity. This type of cutting is used to very good effect whenever a soft, diffused, wispy or fringed edge is desired. Using the razor requires a light versus a heavy-handed approach. In this cut, the razor is used to create softly variegated texture along the edges as opposed to the blunt straight edge achieved with the shear.

APPLY

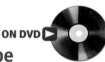
ON DVD ▶

The heavily layered shape will be very light and airy— rounded throughout the interior and contoured close through the nape.

PROCEDURE

1. Comb the hair in natural fall. Take a 1/2" (1.25 cm) section at the front hairline, holding it at low elevation. Cut it to the desired length with the razor. Position the guard toward you and the blade against the hair. Place the razor at that point along the strand where you want to begin the tapering effect. Then etch the razor back and forth along the strand as shown.

2. Cut parallel to the hairline and taper toward your fingers.

3. Continue cutting around the hairline, down the side.

4. Take 1/2" (1.25 cm) partings, position the razor where you want to start tapering the length, and angle it so the section will blend to one you previously cut.

5. Complete the front perimeter on both sides, blending to your initial guide.

6. Refine the fringe all the way around as desired by taking small pieces and razoring them separately. The more pieces you cut, the more light and airy the finished look will be.

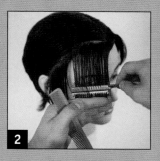

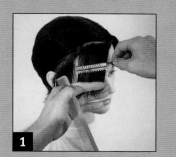

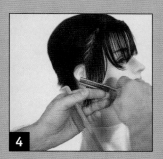

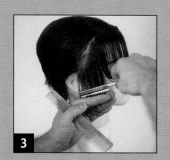

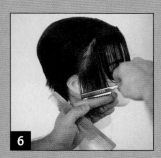

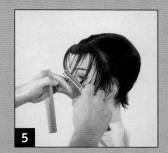

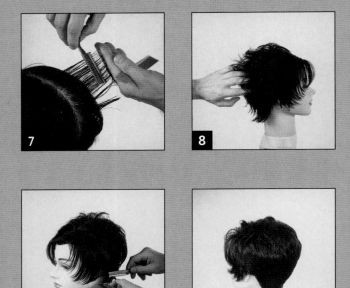

7. Using the previously cut hairline perimeter sections as your traveling guides, work from the front to the back, razoring the hair in 1/2" (1.25 cm) sections. Etch along the top of the hair to taper from the mid-shaft toward the ends, removing the length just above the fingers.

8. Move to the back and taper the nape. Hold the sections slightly outward, then etch along the top surface to create the desired length.

9. The variety of lengths throughout the silhouette creates volume without any hard edges. Personalize the nape area as required. Leave fringed and soft or take short to contrast with the longer frame around the face.

10. The finished style is softly tapered throughout for movement and dimension.

BLOW-DRYING LAYERED RAZOR CUT

OVERVIEW

Razor cutting provides a wide range of opportunity for you to express your artistic and professional talent. It also gives you another way to achieve the ultimate objective: to design a hairstyle that enhances your client's appearance. The key here is the minimal manipulation of the hair. If you blow-dry the hair while moving it in place with your fingers, you'll create a style that truly highlights the detailed texture within the razor cut.

APPLY

With your clients, these technical steps will follow consultation, shampoo, and power or towel drying.

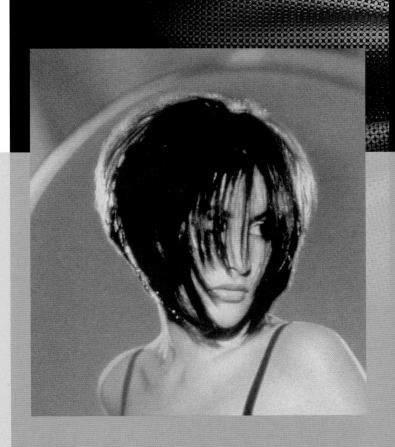

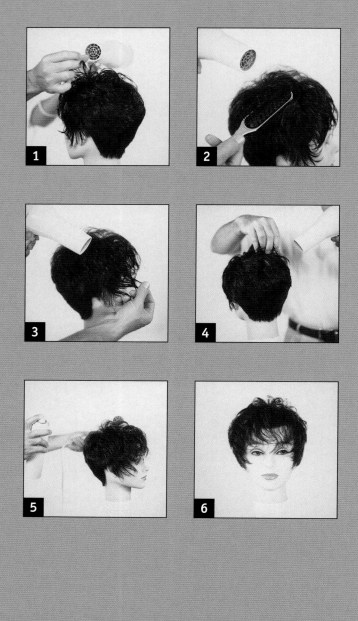

PROCEDURE

1. Apply a styling product of your choice and work it through the hair. Use your fingers and a dryer to gently nudge the textured hair into place. Use your fingertips to separate the textured ends. Notice the massaging action used to add texture and body while drying.

2. Use a small, rubber-based paddle brush to add fullness. In this style the lengths are turned up and forward toward the face.

3. Use a brush around the face to add strength and direction. The brush will add polish to the lengths. Alternate the brush with the fingers to accentuate texture.

4. Use your fingertips to soften and personalize the design.

5. Finish with a combination of spray and blow-dryer for added volume, separation, and texture.

6. The finished style is light and airy with soft fringe-like lengths around the face.

CREATE

Apply this technique to different lengths, colors, and textures for almost endless possibilities.

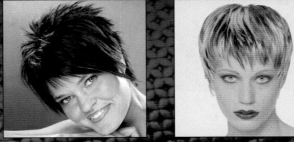
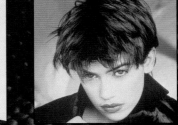
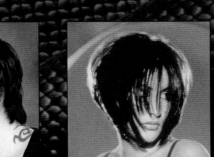

UNIFORM LAYERS

OVERVIEW

In the short uniform cut, the layers you create will echo the curves of the head. The resulting shape is quite sculptural and head hugging. This cut is generally an easy-care, easy-wear design that many of your clients will appreciate.

APPLY

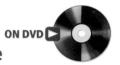
ON DVD

With your clients, these technical steps will follow the consultation and shampoo.

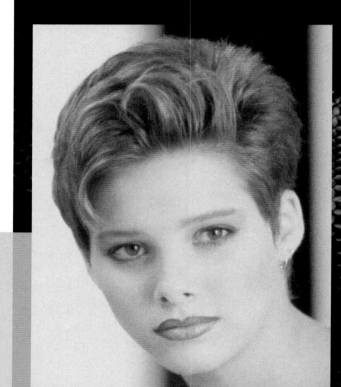

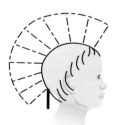

The uniform layered shape consists of equal lengths throughout the entire head. This allows for exceptional movement and volume. You may personalize this cut by the type of frame that you create around the perimeter.

PROCEDURE

1. Comb the hair in natural fall. Part vertically down the center back. Comb out a wide section at the nape with a horizontal part that moves from ear to ear. Starting at the center of the nape, direct and hold a vertical section straight out from the curve of the head and cut it parallel to the curve of the head. This will become your traveling guide.

2. Continue cutting toward the side, using the traveling guide to cut vertical sections. Hold the sections straight out from the curve of the head and cut them parallel to the curve of the head.

3. Cut from the center to the side, then move to the opposite side and cut in the same manner, using a traveling guide, until you reach the perimeter.

4. Move up and release the next horizontal panel. Establish the length by cutting a vertical section at the center, as you did before with the same holding and cutting positions.

5. Move from the center to the left side, then cut from the center to the right side, completing the horizontal section on both sides. Use the traveling guide throughout.

6. Move up to the crown. Part a 1/2" (1.25 cm) vertical section at the center, hold it straight out from the curve of the head, and cut it parallel to the curve of the head to establish the guide for the crown area.

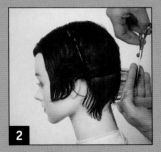

1

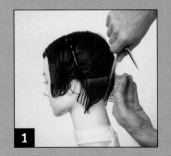

2

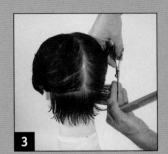

3

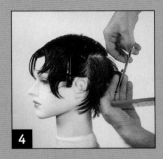

4

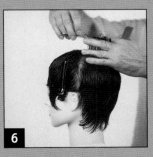

5

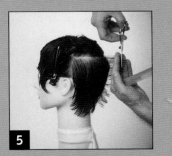

6

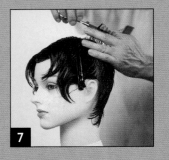

7. From the guide, take radial partings on either side and complete the top, using your initially cut section as a traveling guide. Stop when you reach the point above the ear on each side. Cross-check the back by holding out sections horizontally—the opposite of how you cut them. Clean up any unevenness.

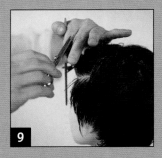

8. Move to the side sections above and in front of the ear. Cut a section at the front side to the same length as the back section. Cut parallel to the curve of the head as you work toward the hairline.

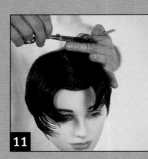
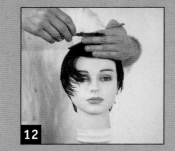

9. Work from just above the ear to the front hairline, then move up to the next section. Cut it in the same manner, holding the hair straight out from the curve of the head.

10. Next, move to the panel along one side of the top. Beginning at the crown area, you now have two guides to follow and blend with—the one from the side crest area and the one from the crown. Part horizontally, direct lengths straight out from the curve of the head, and cut parallel to the head shape.

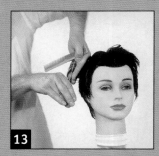

11. Work all the way to the front hairline using the traveling guide. Direct lengths straight out from the curve of the head and cut parallel to the head.

12. Continue in this manner to the front hairline.

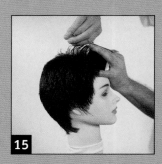
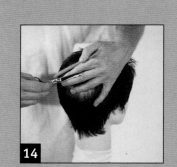

13. Repeat the entire procedure on the other side and top of the head. Work through the center top to blend and ensure balance between the two top panels.

14. Cross-check the hair in every direction, taking partings in the direction opposite to how they were cut.

15. Refine the top and the perimeter as desired.

16. To cut the fringe into a soft, pleasing shape, hold the section out and point cut into the ends with the tips of your scissors. Leave some pieces longer than others.

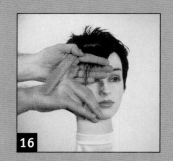

17. Tapering scissors can be used to create longer and shorter lengths along the ends of the hair. Work from the crown area forward to the front hairline. Place the blades into the ends of the hair as controlled by the comb, then methodically work section by section. This will create a well-blended effect.

18. Direct the teeth of the comb downward to hold the hair just behind the ear. Cut around the ear carefully to shape the back hairline.

19. Holding the hair with the comb, cut around the ear from the back, up to the top of the ear.

20. When you reach the top, cut the hair in front of the ear by angling your scissors downward.

21. Refine the line around the ear and in front of it.

22. Use a scissors-over-comb technique to diagonally work upward from the perimeter hairline toward the center back.

23. Then reverse and work diagonally from the center back to the area behind the ear to blend and cross-check lengths while creating the shape.

24. To taper in the nape area, comb the hair at a diagonal and cut, using the scissors-over-comb technique. Then move in the opposite diagonal direction upward from the center back toward the ear area to blend and cross-check lengths. The finished cut provides a soft, wispy perimeter frame around the face, and the extra length through the crown complements and harmonizes with the short nape area.

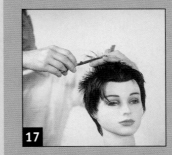

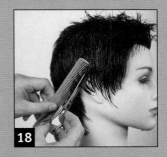

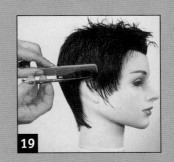

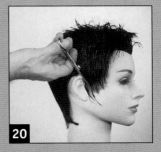

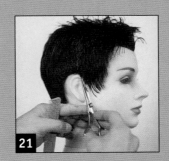

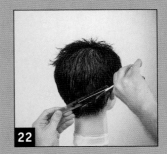

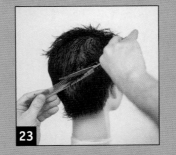

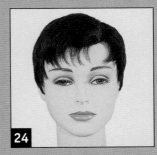

CREATE

Apply this technique to different lengths, colors, and textures for almost endless possibilities.

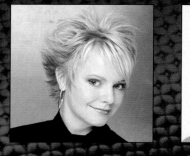
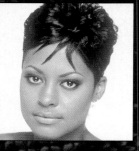
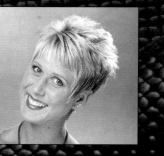
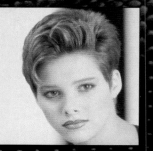

MEN'S HAIRCUTTING

LONG LAYER

OVERVIEW

With this first men's haircut, you will learn how to create designs by producing a more squared shape. As you remember from the women's haircutting part of this program, shapes for females are more rounded and curved. Men's shapes generally have more definite and squared weight areas.

The procedures you'll use with men's cuts come from classical men's barbering techniques, and they'll serve you well in the salon. For example, with this long layer haircut, you will learn how and why to hold your hands in certain positions as you work around the head. Holding the hair straight out will allow you to achieve the desired layered effect while keeping longer lengths. At the same time, you are creating a definite style and design for the male client, not

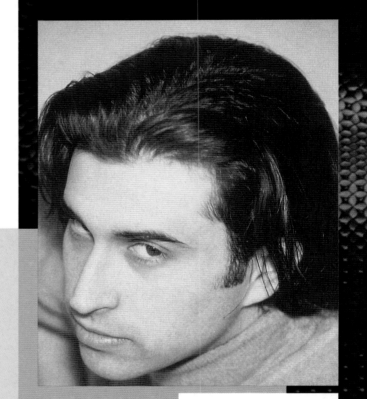

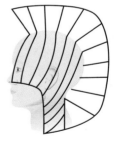

This long layered silhouette provides textural movement and dimension. The layers begin at the nose level and progress to the collar-length perimeter.

just removing uneven ends. Another example is cutting in the palm of your hand; this allows you to better see what you're cutting, as well as create a flatter surface to cut on for more control.

Another method introduced with this haircut is cutting the sideburn area with a scissors-over-comb technique. In this technique, you use the comb to hold the hair in place while you use the tips of your scissors to remove the lengths. This requires a steady hand and close attention to what you're doing. For men's designs, sideburns play a key role in the total look.

Men's haircutting techniques use scissors with longer cutting blades. These allow you to remove more hair at a time and are also necessary for the fine tapering techniques often used in the nape area of shorter haircuts. The haircutting comb has both fine-spaced and wide-spaced teeth, which are used for shorter and longer lengths of hair. The spacing of the teeth will adjust the tension for cutting.

APPLY

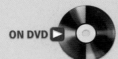 ON DVD ▶

With your clients, these technical steps will follow consultation and shampoo.

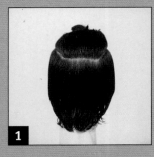

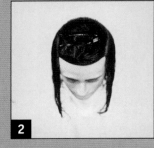

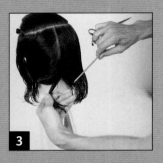

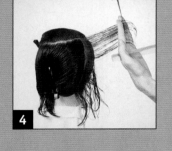

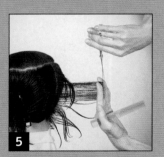

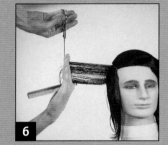

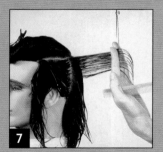

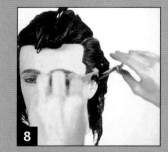

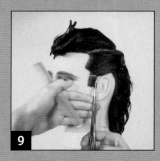

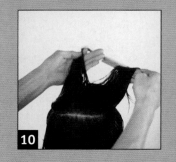

PROCEDURE

1. Begin this haircut by parting off the lower section from the top section using a horseshoe-shaped parting.

2. Use the recession areas at the front hairline and the crown as your guidelines.

3. Take a vertical section that moves from the top of the back area to the center of the nape. This section, when cut, will be your traveling guide for the entire haircut. Use small sections throughout the cut to ensure an even length balance.

4. Comb the section straight out from the back of the head. Establish the length to be removed and cut your traveling guide.

5. Cut from the top of the section to the bottom, working toward the nape of the neck.

6. Continue parting vertical sections, holding them straight out from the side of the head and cutting vertically as you work around the head. Use the traveling guide as you cut until you reach the front hairline.

7. Return to the center back of the head and pick up your initial guide. Use it to cut the opposite side in the same manner, taking small sections and working toward the opposite side of the head. Again, stop when you reach the hairline.

8. To cut the sideburn, comb and clip the hair above it out of the way, exposing the sideburn section. Establish the desired length and cut. Then use a scissors-over-comb technique to remove excess fullness from the sideburn.

9. Detail the perimeter of the sideburn using a freehand technique. Use your opposite hand to stabilize as you cut.

10. Unclip the hair on the top. Take a center part that moves from the back of the head to the front.

11. To cut the top section, take a horizontal parting at the back of the section that moves from the center to the right side of the head.

12. Use the previously cut exterior as your guide. Be certain to hold the hair straight out from the head as you cut out and, in this instance, parallel to the head.

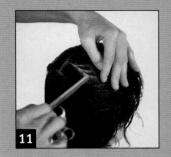
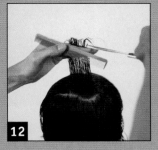

13. Work toward the front, horizontally parting out small sections and cutting to the established length. Notice that each section of hair is directed straight out from the head. Be certain not to overdirect any of your partings.

14. When you reach the front hairline, move to the back of the section and cut the left side of the top, using the same technique.

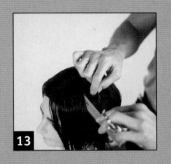
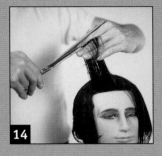

15., 16. For a natural finished look, apply the desired liquid styling product, then finger style the hair.

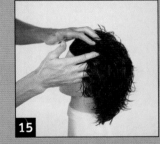
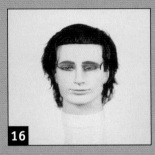

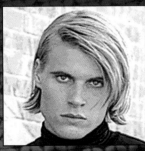
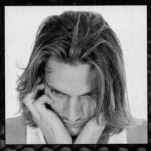

CREATE

Apply this technique to different lengths, colors, and textures for almost endless possibilities.

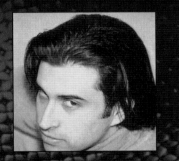

OVERVIEW

This haircut begins with the longer-length haircut you just created. You will not be removing a great deal of length—just enough to create a medium-length layered shape. You will establish a long length guide using facial features as reference points. By holding the hair in a vertical position when you cut and not moving it away from its parting, you have greater control because you have a more accurate length to work with. Because this is a traveling guide, pay close attention to the sizes of sections that you take. For accuracy, part out smaller- or medium-sized sections, 1/4 to 1/2 inch, and use the end of your cutting comb that has wider-spaced teeth. You will cut on the the back and inside of your hand. You'll be creating a squared shape to accentuate and

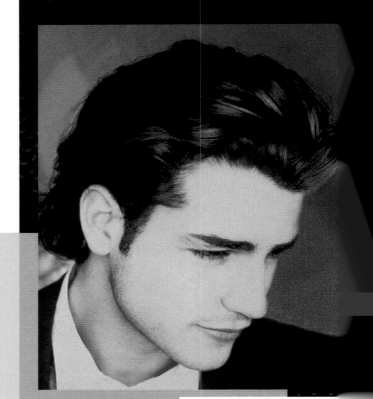

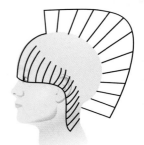

The layered effect in this shape is created by cutting the entire perimeter to a mid-length traveling guide. This blends with the interior lengths that are cut to build weight around the crest area.

complement the male head shape.
Avoid creating a curved or rounded
shape as you cut by keeping the head
in an upright position.

APPLY

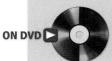

ON DVD

**With your clients, these
technical steps will follow
consultation and shampoo.**

PROCEDURE

1. Establish the length for the cut by using a reference point on the face. Once established, this length will be the guide for the remainder of the cut.

2. Take a vertical section through the center top of the head. Hold the hair straight out and cut parallel to the head.

3. Use this length as a guide and continue cutting the center section, working toward the crown and following the curvature of the head.

4. Now, section off the top of the head from the crown to both recession areas at the front hairline.

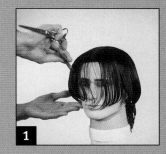

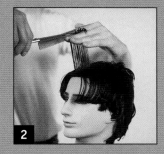

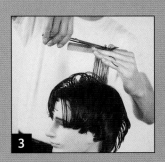

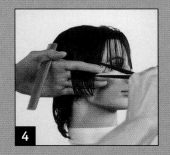

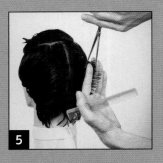

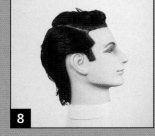

5. Moving to the back, vertically part down the center and continue establishing the length from the crown to the nape of the neck by cutting vertically. This will be your guide for the entire back section.

6. Continue through the back using this technique.

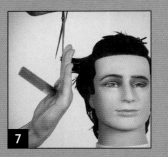

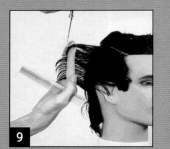

7. Work from the center back to the front hairline, continuing to cut vertical sections to your traveling guide.

8. The completed side should blend neatly. Cross-check horizontally where needed.

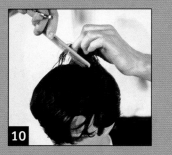

9. Return to the guide at the center back and cut the left side all the way to the front hairline, continuing to use the same technique.

10. Moving to the top section, unclip the hair and comb it forward. Take a horizontal parting across the top at the back of the section.

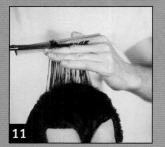

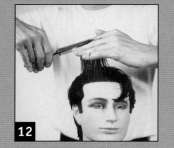

11. Comb and hold the hair straight out from the top of the head and cut, using the previously cut section from the top center as your guide.

12. Continue cutting the top section, taking small partings as you move from the crown to the front hairline. To ensure the desired layered effect, use consistency in the holding, cutting, and scissors positions. Upon finishing the cut, comb through the lengths to check the cut response. Cross-check vertically as needed.

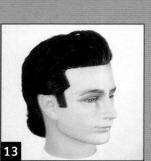

13. The backswept lengths are easily achieved in this haircut with the internal layers that flow over the perimeter graduation.

CREATE

Apply this technique to different lengths, colors, and textures for almost endless possibilities.

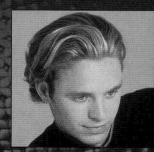

SHORT LAYER

OVERVIEW

You are preparing to cut to a shorter length. As with the two previous haircuts, you will begin by establishing the traveling length guide. Begin at the back of the head and work your way toward the face. Because you are cutting the lengths shorter, your hands will be closer to the head. Note that you will want to avoid resting your hands against the head as you cut so you are able to control the cutting angles. When you hold the sections straight out relative to the head area being cut, don't overdirect them forward or back. By holding them straight out, the accuracy of your cutting will remain constant.

APPLY

With your clients, these technical steps will follow the consultation and shampoo.

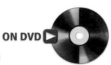

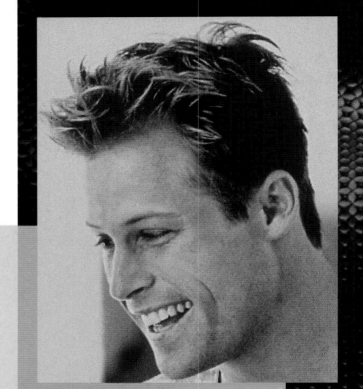

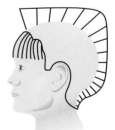

This silhouette provides a closely tapered perimeter hairline to combine with the short internal layers.

PROCEDURE

1. Sectioning off the top, start at the round of the head in the back and work toward the recession area on both sides at the front. At the back, take a 1/2" (1.25 cm) vertical section down the center back all the way to the nape.

2. Hold the section straight out from the back of the head and cut vertically from the top to the nape. This will be your traveling guide for the rest of the haircut. Starting next to the guide section, work vertically, taking 1/2" (1.25 cm) sections as you move around the back area of the head.

3. Leave the sideburn section free for now.

4. Return to the center back to cut the opposite side of the head. Pick up the traveling guide; sweep it over to each new section being cut. Make sure that the traveling guide is visible at all times. Work around the head toward the front hairline.

5. Establish the length of the sideburn.

6. Use a scissors-over-comb technique to remove bulk around the ear. This will create a nice, clean look all around the ear. Cut both sideburns in the same manner.

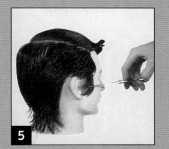

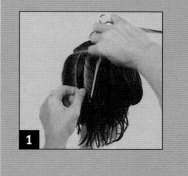

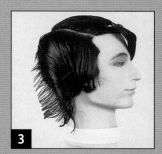

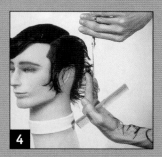

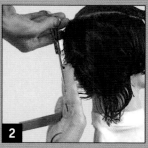

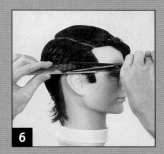

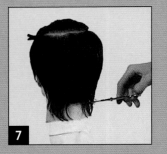

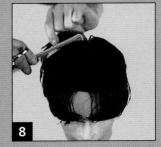

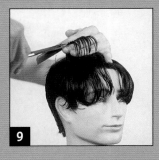

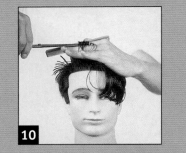

7. Establish the length at the nape of the neck and cut both sides of the nape horizontally.

8. To complete the cut, move to the top area, which was previously sectioned out. Take a horizontal parting that moves from the center of the back of the section to the right side of the head.

9. Use the previously cut lengths from the crest area as a guide, making certain to hold the hair straight out from the curve of the head. Cut parallel to the curve of the head.

10. Continue cutting small, horizontal sections to the guide as you work toward the front hairline. Be certain not to overdirect any of your partings. When you reach the front hairline, repeat the cutting technique on the left side of the top section.

11. The lengths of the finished haircut blend perfectly when the hair is combed back. The finished style highlights the precise layers created in this shape.

CREATE

Apply this technique to
different lengths, colors,
and textures for almost
endless possibilities.

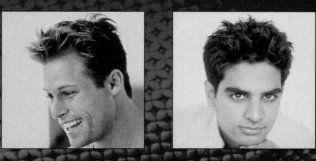

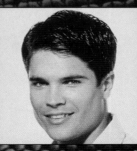

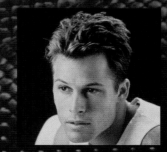

LONG GRADUATION

OVERVIEW

This long graduation cut creates more fullness than you've created in the previous two haircuts because you use no close tapering or fade techniques. Working with your scissors, you will create a graduation of balanced lengths throughout. Note that the techniques used in this graduation cut will remove considerable bulk even though the finished look sports a full amount of volume. The main key to this haircut is using exact elevation angles.

APPLY

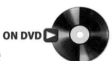
ON DVD

With your clients, these technical steps will follow consultation and shampoo.

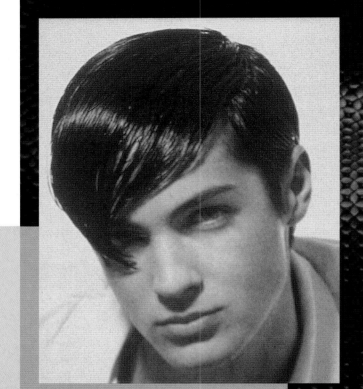

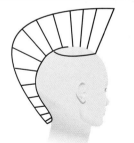

The long graduation is the classic silhouette for the male client who desires longer hair. Lengths graduate upward toward the crest area, where a concentration of weight is located.

PROCEDURE

1. Part off a section at the round of the head, as shown. Clip this top section out of the way.

2. Comb the hair straight down and cut a blunt perimeter line around the head. The comb is used to control the lengths and create the cut line. Make certain you have a clean, balanced perimeter length all around the head.

3. Move to the back and take a vertical section down the center of the head. Elevate and hold the hair straight out from the back of the head and cut in diagonally, using the perimeter as your guide.

4. Continue cutting vertical sections, working from the center of the back toward the front. Return to the center back and continue working through the opposite side. Cut all the way to the front hairline.

5. Clean up the sideburn as needed.

6. Unclip the top section and part horizontally through the side, moving from the back to the front hairline.

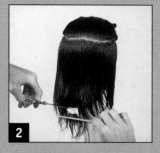

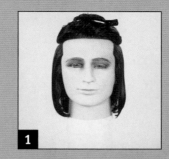

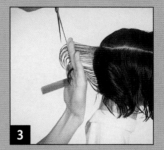

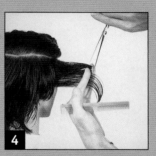

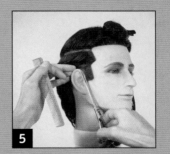

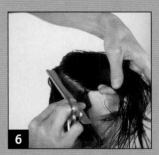

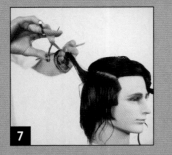
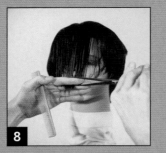

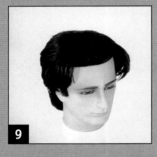

7. Using the previously cut exterior length as your guide, direct the hair straight out from the curve of the head and cut to the guide. Use this procedure from the back of the section all the way through to the sides. Continue cutting small sections until you run out of hair.

8. Comb the hair down in the front and cut to the lip line to refine the front perimeter line.

9. The hair has been styled to accentuate the graduated effect. This graduation may be adapted according to the client's needs and desires.

> **Magic is believing in yourself, if you can do that, you can make anything happen.**
>
> *Foka Gomez*

CREATE

Apply this technique to different lengths, colors, and textures for almost endless possibilities.

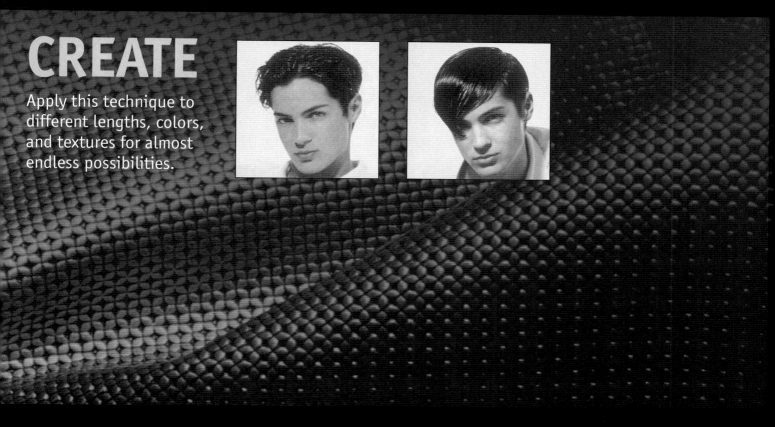

MEDIUM GRADUATED TAPER

OVERVIEW

This design emphasizes volume in the crown area, with a more closely tapered look on the sides and in the back. New to you with this haircut will be parting the hair horizontally, elevating it at a consistent angle throughout the crest area of the head, and creating a balanced form. Along with cutting with your fingers in a vertical position, you will also hold your hands and fingers in horizontal positions. You'll see results of these techniques in the weight line that you create around the crest area.

APPLY

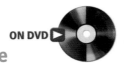

With your clients, these technical steps will follow consultation and shampoo.

This silhouette is extremely popular with male clientele. Longer graduated interval lengths contrast with the short tapered exterior lengths. This is a truly versatile shape that can be styled in a number of ways.

PROCEDURE

1. Part off a section at the round of the head, using the points of recession at the front hairline and the crown of the head as guidelines.

2. Begin by taking a vertical parting at the center of the back of the head from the crown to the nape.

3. Hold each section out from the head and cut in diagonally. This will be your guide for the entire perimeter area. Continue taking vertical partings and cutting to the traveling guide as you work toward the front. Repeat on both sides.

4. Move to the nape and use your comb to hold the hair, resting it against the head at an angle. Cut the hair at the neckline. Work across the comb to cut, then blend upward with a freehand clipper technique, using a light and meticulous touch.

5. To finish the bottom of the hairline, cut freehand, using a clipper rocking technique.

6. To graduate short lengths around the ear, rest the base of the comb on an angle from the hairline outward. Run the clipper lengthwise along the comb.

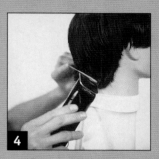
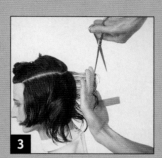
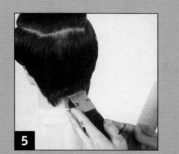
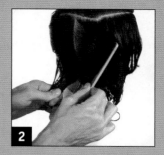
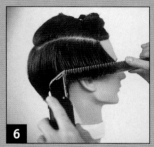
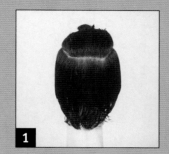

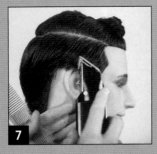

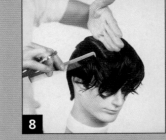

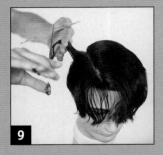

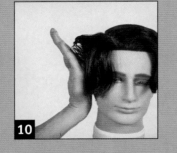

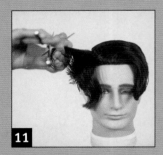

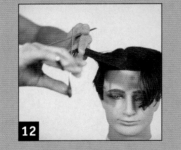

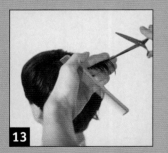

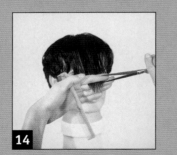

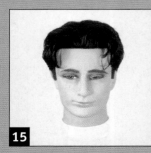

7. Hold the blade of the clippers at an angle as you trim around the ear.

8. Comb the interior hair forward and down. To cut the top, take a horizontal parting as you move from the back to the front. The partings should be small enough to ensure an even length throughout the top.

9. Using the length from the crest as your stable guide, comb the section of hair up to the guide, which should be held straight out from the head.

10. Notice the graduated angle as well as the diminished weight at the crest from using the outlined cutting technique.

11. Continue taking horizontal partings, directing the hair out from the crest area, and cutting. Work from the perimeter of the top section to the center and from back to front. Hold the hair straight out from the crest of the head. This becomes increasingly important as you move toward the front hairline.

12. Upon completing this area, repeat the process in the opposite top side area.

13. Blend the lengths at the back of the head by directing the hair back to the graduated exterior guide. The elevation or holding position used here is consistent with the method used for the sides.

14. Comb the hair around the face forward and cut the entire front hairline section, blending it to create a clean line at the front.

15. The finished graduated taper is symmetrical in nature. The longer weight area throughout the interior provides length for styling versatility, yet the short perimeter hairline is precisely contoured for a clean, refined look.

CREATE

Apply this technique to different lengths, colors, and textures for almost endless possibilities.

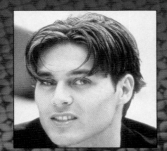 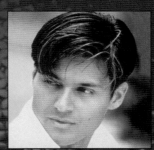

LAYERS OVER SHORT GRADUATED TAPER

OVERVIEW

This design uses the technique of graduation on shorter lengths than the previous haircut and involves cutting with a combination of scissors and clippers. Clippers are frequently used for cutting men's hair because they allow for quick cutting and close cropping of the hair around the sides, the ears, and at the nape. They also work well in the clipper-over-comb technique, which is highly controlled.

Because you can remove a large amount of hair with the clipper blades, you will need to gain expertise through continued practice so you do not remove too much when you cut. You can return to any area of the head to remove more length, if need be.

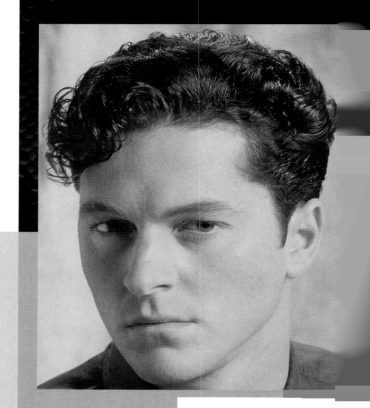

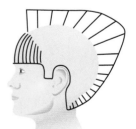

In this silhouette a closely tapered perimeter progresses into the layered interior. The interior length allows for great versatility in the styling, while the closely tapered perimeter creates a contoured effect.

APPLY

ON DVD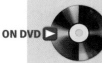

With your clients, these technical steps will follow consultation and shampoo.

PROCEDURE

1. Section off the hair at the round of the head, using the recession areas at the front and the crown of the head as guidelines.

2. Start at the front temple on one side of the head, taking a 1/2" (1.25 cm) vertical section. This will be cut to become your traveling guide. Direct the lengths straight out from the side of the head and position the fingers diagonally. Cut in diagonally to create the desired length. Continue taking vertical partings as you work your way back.

3. Once you pass the ear, extend the guide from the top to the nape of the neck as you move around the head.

4. Cut to your traveling guide, continuing to hold the hair straight out as you go. Work all the way around to the temple area on the opposite side.

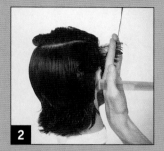

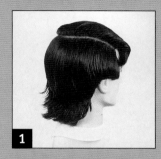

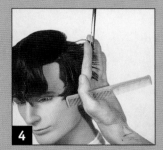

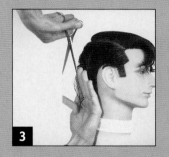

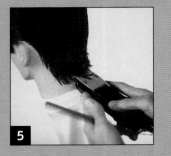

5

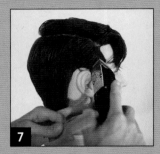

6

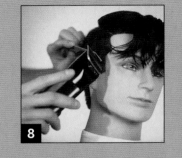

7

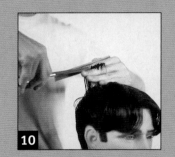

8

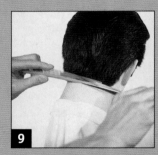

9

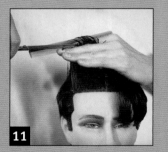

10

11

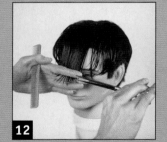

12

5. Change to the clippers and begin cutting at the center of the nape with the blade resting against the head. Notice how the two hands are holding the clippers for steadiness and balance. As you move up into the hairline, slowly rock the clippers away from the round of the head. Repeat the cutting technique throughout the entire nape area.

6. Taper the sides next. Blend freehand at the lower hairline area, then use a comb to pick up the hair behind the ear and cut. Notice that the previously cut hair in the comb acts as your guide. The comb and scissors must move together.

7. Holding the clippers at an angle, continue to cut the outline around the ear. This will create a nice, smooth line around the ear. Notice the angle of the blades against the head.

8. With the comb held at an angle and the base of the comb resting against the head, cut the hair by moving the clippers across the comb. Your previously cut vertical sections will be your guide for the angle at which you should hold the comb.

9. Refine the neckline and entire perimeter using the barbering comb or a tapering comb. The taper comb will create the closest possible degrees of taper around the perimeter, given the narrowness of the comb and the narrow-spaced teeth.

10. Starting at the back top of the head, cut the top section. Take a horizontal parting that moves from the center to the right side of the head. Using the previously cut vertical section as your guide, hold the hair straight out from the head, then cut toward the center top.

11. Work from the back of the section to the hairline, then repeat the technique on the left side of the head.

12. Comb the hair down onto the face and connect the front section of the fringe across the front. Be sure to cut the hairline in front of the temple to blend in with the fringe.

13. Add the finishing touch. Brush and place the lengths of hair for a well-balanced shape. If desired, mist through the top area with a light-hold finishing spray.

14. This sophisticated style is a perennial favorite among male clients. It is neat, controlled, and well groomed in its expression.

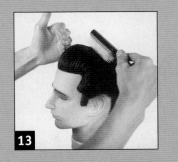

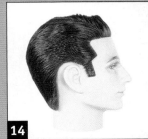

CREATE

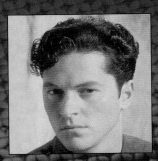

Apply this technique to different lengths, colors, and textures for almost endless possibilities.

OVERVIEW

This classic, tapered haircut brings you to another level of expertise as you learn how to apply the razor within men's cutting. As you've seen so far, each cutting tool is chosen to produce exact results. Although the razor is not used throughout this entire haircut, it will create finely detailed transitions between areas around the perimeter hairline, as well as blend the ends through the interior. Working with the razor will give you new options for future haircutting and personalizing haircuts for clients with many kinds of hair types. Working with scissors, clippers, and a razor helps you create a popular yet timeless look that will always be in demand.

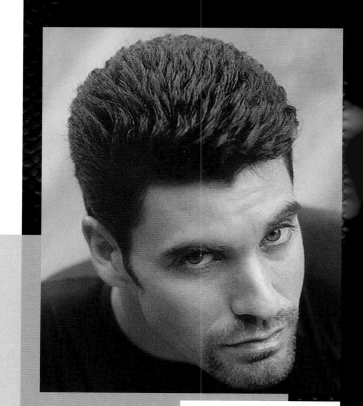

This shape features a dynamic tapered perimeter that progresses into the squared silhouette in the interior. The weight area in this cut is around the crest area.

APPLY

ON DVD ▶
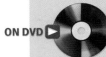

With your clients, these technical steps will follow consultation and shampoo.

PROCEDURE

1. Part off a section at the round of the head, using the recession areas at the front hairline and the crown of the head as guidelines.

2. Part a vertical section that moves down the center back to the nape of the neck. Direct and hold lengths straight out from the back of the head. Cut to the fingers, which are held in a precise, vertical position. Cut the vertical section all the way down to the nape. The shape as influenced by the cutting position will feature a weight buildup around the crest area.

3. Continue to take vertical partings as you move toward the side; cut from the top of the parting all the way to the nape.

4. Take small, clean sections to ensure an even length throughout the exterior area.

5. When you reach the front hairline, return to the center back and use the same technique to cut the opposite side of the head.

6. Moving to the back nape area, use a clipper-over-comb technique and cut in a low taper. Place the base of the cutting comb against the hairline area and angle the comb out, as clippering lengths creates a smooth, even, tapered closeness between the hairline and vertically cut hair.

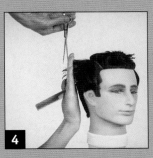

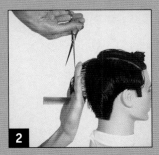

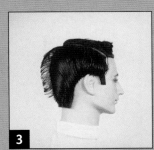

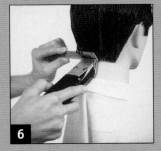

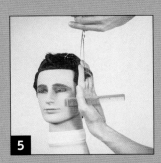

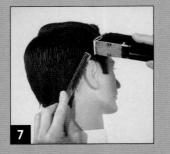

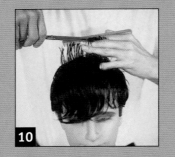

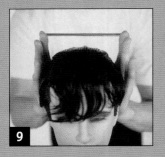

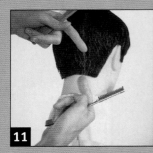

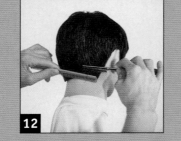

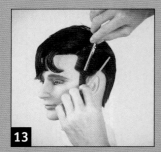

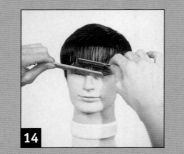

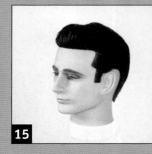

7. Continue this tapering technique all the way around the perimeter to the front of the head.

8. Next, angle the clippers around the ear to make a cleanly cut line around it.

9. Moving to the top crown area, comb and hold the hair straight up from the top of the head for cutting horizontally. This will ensure a square shape. Using the previously cut exterior lengths as your guide, take horizontally sections across the top of the head and cut horizontally to the guide.

10. Continue working toward the front until all the hair is cut. Direct and hold the lengths straight up from the top of the head and cut to the horizontal traveling guide.

11. Use the razor with a guard on and the blade against the hair to blend the transition area. The comb and razor rotate to control and cut the hair.

12. Use the comb to control the hair and hold the blade at a medium angle as you run it through the hair to reduce any weight buildup. Work down toward the nape.

13. Repeat the razoring technique all around the perimeter, maintaining an even amount of pressure and a consistent angle. A light touch is to be used with this technique to avoid removing too much hair. Use light strokes when personalizing the area around the ear.

14. Use extra caution as you remove excess weight in the front fringe area. By removing weight here, you'll have more control in styling the hair.

15. Notice the clean lines in the finished look.

CREATE

Apply this technique to different lengths, colors, and textures for almost endless possibilities.

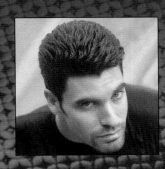 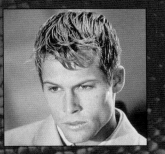 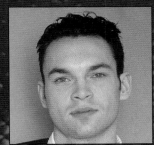

HIGH TAPER

OVERVIEW

This highly tapered men's haircut uses very short graduation cutting techniques to create a "fade" look. This means that the hair is very closely cut, with the scalp showing in the perimeter areas. At the same time, the overall finish of this cut shows smooth transitions from very short to somewhat longer lengths in the crown for styling freedom. Here the focus is on using scissors, clippers, and both types of cutting combs to produce specific results. With each haircut, you are seeing how you need accuracy and increased skill to produce these carefully planned and cut designs. With shorter lengths of hair, the planning of the haircut and the application of the techniques become very important. The balance of the shape and how well it complements the

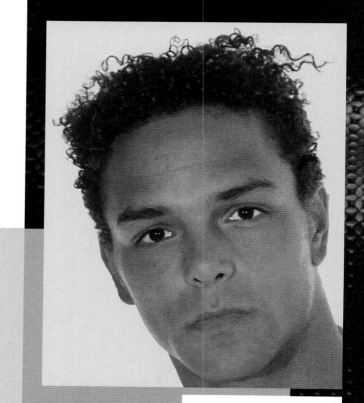

The dramatic "fade" around the perimeter can be progressive and edgy or classic in nature. The tight perimeter progresses into the longer internal lengths.

client's head shape and facial features are really the keys to the success of your efforts. With your increasing experience, your eye will tell you if a cut is proportionate for the client.

APPLY

ON DVD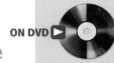

With your clients, these technical steps will follow consultation and shampoo.

PROCEDURE

1. Part off a section at the round of the head, using the recession areas and the crown as guidelines. Moving to the nape of the neck, start cutting in the middle using the clippers. Move up against the head and slowly rock the clippers away from the round of the head. This section will be your guide for the entire perimeter.

2. Work from the center of the nape to the side. When you reach the side perimeter, move the clippers parallel to the hairline while cutting.

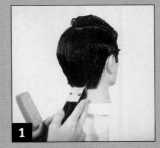

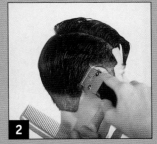

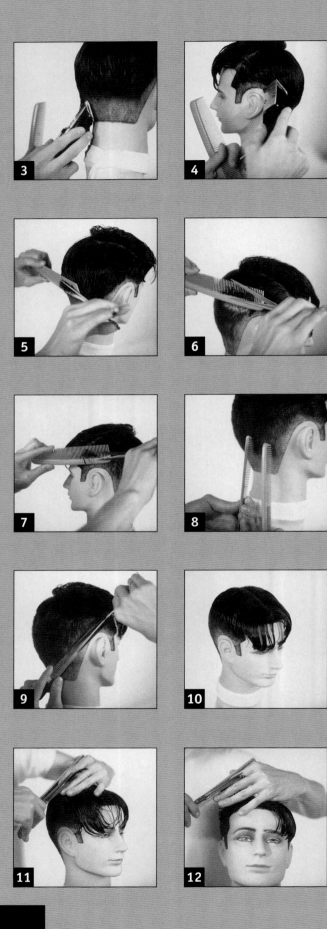

3. Now cut the other side, restarting at the center nape and working toward the front of the head. Be certain to maintain an even amount of pressure while working with the clippers. Cut each section to the same length as the previous one before you move on to another section.

4. When the perimeter hairline is complete, hold the clippers at an angle and cut a clean line around the ear. This makes a smooth finish around the hairline. Repeat on the other side.

5., 6. Using a larger cutting comb and scissors, start at the center nape of the neck and continue to cut the hair to the established perimeter length. Be certain to work consistently from section to section, up to the top crown area of the head. Work straight upward through the back of the head using the scissors-over-comb technique.

7. Continue working to the front of the head, using the previously cut hair as a guide. Complete one side, then cut the opposite side, starting at the center nape and working toward the front.

8. Use the tapering comb to finish the hairline at the back and sides. The length of hair you're removing in this process is very small, but it will make the finished results perfect. This type of comb makes it very easy to work closely around the perimeter hairline.

9. Taper in this transition area all the way around the perimeter hairline.

10. Comb the top forward and divide the top section in half by taking a center parting that moves down the middle of the head.

11., 12. Moving to the crown, take a horizontal parting that moves from the center to the right side of the head. Using the exterior cut section as your guide, cut the hair, working toward the center top of the head. Continue cutting small partings as you work toward the front of the head. Direct lengths straight out and cut diagonally to the traveling guide. After you cut your last section at the recession area, shift the final partings back to this guide.

13. Repeat the procedure on the opposite side of the head. Using the first guide established at the crown and the perimeter guide on the side, cut the hair between the two guides. Work from the back of the section toward the hairline, remembering to shift the final partings.

14. When you've completed the second side, comb the front fringe lengths forward and cut the hair from the shorter sides straight across the front. To finish, apply the appropriate product and style into the desired shape.

15. Here, the hair is styled asymmetrically.

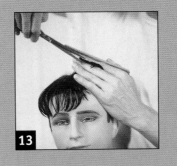
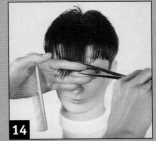
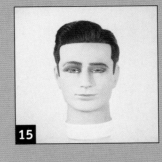

CREATE

Apply this technique to different lengths, colors, and textures for almost endless possibilities.

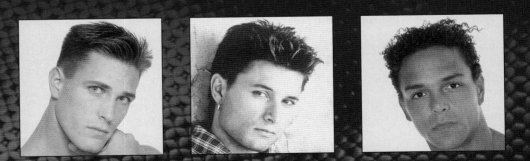

SHORT BRUSH CUT

OVERVIEW

With this men's haircut, you will learn the shortest graduation technique, which produces shorter lengths at the nape progressing to longer lengths at the top of the head. This is a versatile and popular design because it allows the comfort and ease of short hair while offering a longer length interior.

You'll want to fine-tune your scissors-over-comb coordination, which you'll need to master for this haircutting technique. There are fewer partings, so you must have extra control as you cut in a freehand style. You'll use the scissors-over-comb technique both to create a finely tapered effect throughout the exterior area of the head and to hold longer internal lengths out from the head to cut. Thus, this one

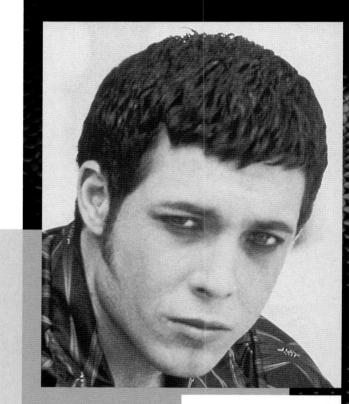

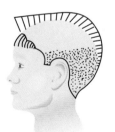

This short, dynamic shape features closely graduated lengths through the interior that progress into longer interval lengths that echo the curve of the head.

technique produces a pair of distinct effects seen in the contrasting lengths of hair. The combination of haircutting techniques and shapes created opens new possibilities for designing as you master your skills.

APPLY

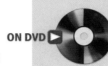
ON DVD ▷

With your clients, these technical steps will follow consultation and shampoo.

PROCEDURE

1. Use a pie-shaped parting to section off the top, from the center crown to the front recession area on both sides.

2. Note the combing and holding of the large-toothed cutting comb for working upward through the back area.

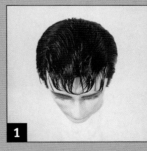

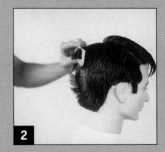

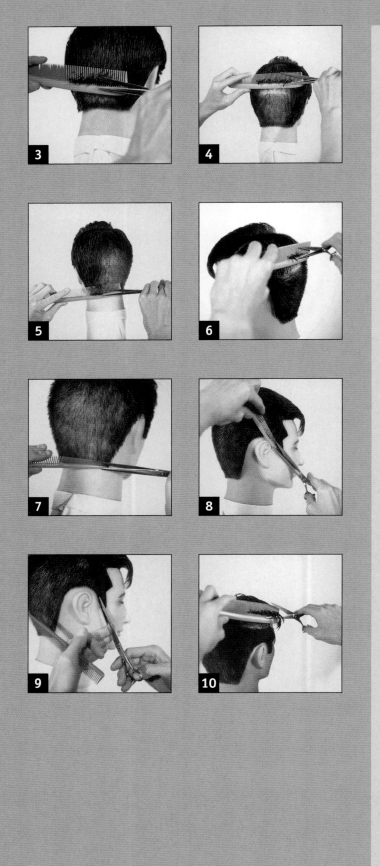

3. Begin cutting at the center of the nape of the neck, using a scissors-over-comb technique.

4. Continue with your scissors-over-comb cutting until the hair is the length that you want. Do not move onto the next section until you have established the desired length and the hair is even; this will be your guide for the entire cut. Once the length is established, work toward the right side and continue using a scissors-over-comb technique. Complete the entire side, making certain that there are no lines of unevenness in the hair.

5. Return to the center of the nape and use the previously established length as your guide. Feed the hair through the base of your comb and cut the hair precisely when it passes through the base.

6. It is very important to hold the still blade stationary and at the base of the comb when you cut. (Use your thumb to move the cutting blade only.) Work toward the left and complete the side as before.

7. Use a barbering or tapered comb to create the final details of the finished taper. When you're cutting with a tapered comb, use the same procedure and technique that you used with the large-toothed comb.

8. The tapered comb allows you to get the hair shorter and closer at the lower part of the perimeter hairline and makes cutting the nape, the sideburns, and the ear area easier.

9. To detail around the sideburns, use a freehand technique and the blade tips of your scissors.

10. Using your large-toothed cutting comb, begin cutting through the crest area and top, using a scissors-over-comb technique. First, comb the hair up from the side until you see the guide from the perimeter hairline feed into the base of the comb. As you continue to work upward toward the center top, use the previously cut section as your guide.

11. Incorporate the front with the length on the sides. Work from one side upward through the center top, and repeat on opposite side.

12. Move to the front hairline and work toward the crown, using the same cutting technique to blend the entire top.

13. In the finished, short brush cut, all the hair blends evenly. This cut is styled here for a more accentuated and piecy texture effect.

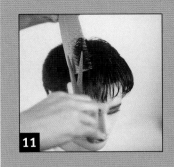

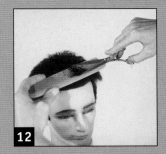

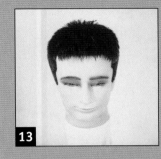

CREATE

Apply this technique to different lengths, colors, and textures for almost endless possibilities.

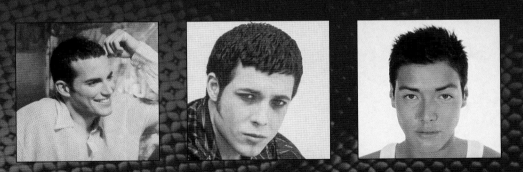

CONTEMPORARY TAPER

OVERVIEW

In this cut, you will use your tapering techniques to fashion a medium-length look that sports volume, versatility, and finishing options. Paying close attention to detail work throughout this haircut results in a smooth finish that is sure to please. A closely tapered neckline progresses to increasingly longer lengths through the interior for volume and height. You will create this design by using your scissors and clippers with a variety of techniques to both remove length and create detailed work.

APPLY

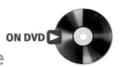
ON DVD ▶

With your clients, these technical steps will follow consultation and shampoo.

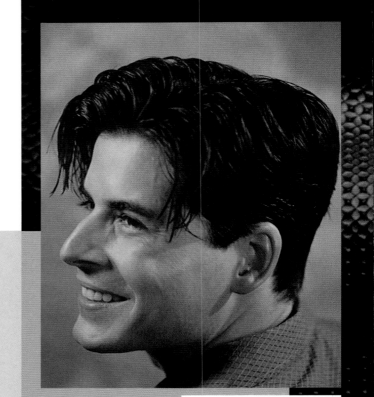

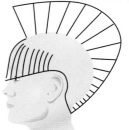

This cut is close and sculptured around the perimeter hairline, progressing to longer lengths through the interior.

PROCEDURE

1. Part off a section at the round of the head, using the recession areas at the front hairline and the crown as your guidelines.

2. Begin at the center back, just below the sectioned-off crown area. Take a vertical section, shift the hair diagonally up and out from the head, and cut vertically. Be sure to maintain consistency in the holding and cutting positions along with even tension when working toward the sides. Repeat on the opposite back side of the head.

3. At the crown, release a diagonal section and cut to the guide length. Continue to release diagonal settings, direct lengths straight out from the side of the head, and cut. Bring the hair straight out from the side of the head and angle the fingers slightly to the line that increases in length from the crest area. Angle the fingers diagonally for cutting toward the front hairline. Use this technique to the center top.

4. Repeat this procedure on the opposite side of the head.

5. At the center crown area, check and blend the lengths from the two panels that were cut through the top.

6. Take horizontal sections across the top of the head. Hold the hair straight out and round off any unevenness through the center as you work toward the front hairline.

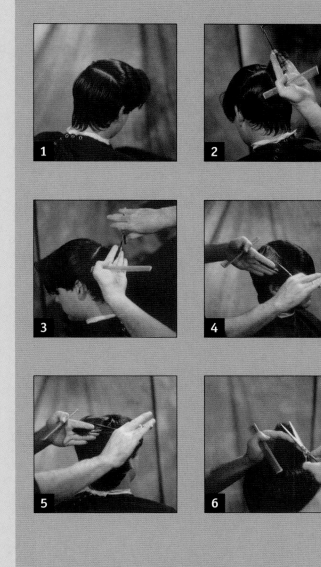

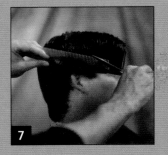

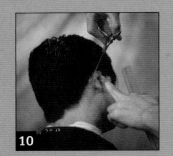

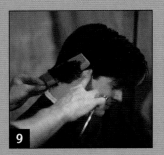

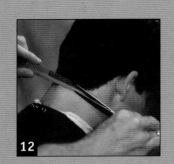

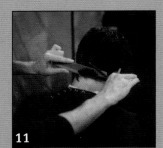

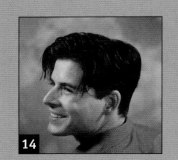

7. Use a scissors-over-comb technique to remove any bulk and weight around the ear. Notice the angle at which the comb is held.

8. Refine the line around the ear, using your scissors in a freehand technique as you outline the ear.

9. Use a scissors-over-comb technique to taper the perimeter sides toward the nape. This ensures a smooth, clean look. It is very important to move your scissors and the comb in unison. Note how the ear is held out of the way.

10. Again, refine and detail the perimeter line.

11. When both perimeter sides are complete, remove bulk at the nape with your scissors and a comb.

12. Detail and refine the taper of the nape using a small barbering comb. Note the fine detailing that you can achieve.

13. To complete the haircut, use a clipper to refine any extra hair around the neck and sides.

14. In the finished look, there is enough length in front for a variety of styling options.

CREATE

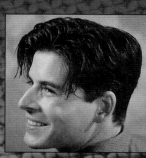

Apply this technique to
different lengths, colors,
and textures for almost
endless possibilities.

GENTLEMAN'S TAPER

OVERVIEW

This shorter tapered look is ideal for the well-groomed businessman who prefers shorter lengths but still wants enough length for styling choices. This look converts easily from a recreational to a professional setting for an always-groomed image. It would work well for several different face shapes and hair textures, including naturally curly or wavy hair. Note that no area is cut too short or extreme; instead the look projects a well-designed image, a result of precision cutting based on the understanding of cutting techniques.

APPLY

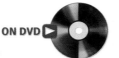 ON DVD ▶

With your clients, these technical steps will follow consultation and shampoo.

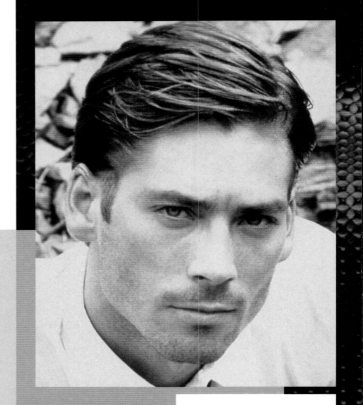

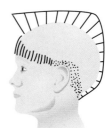

This heavily layered and tapered cut features a slight elongation through the top and around the fringe area for adaptability.

PROCEDURE

1. Establish a section at the round of the head, using the recession areas at the front hairline and the crown of the head as your guidelines. Start above the ear. Take a vertical section, hold the hair straight out from the head, and cut.

2. Work from the ear to the front hairline, shifting the last section at the front hairline back to slightly increase the length. This will allow extra length to personalize the fringe area, particularly when the front hairline is receding.

3. Vertically part out sections, holding straight out from the head. Cut parallel to the head. Move to the panel above the ear and cut to blend with the previously cut section. Continue through the center back. Repeat on the other side.

4. Take horizontal sections through the interior from the center top to the outside of the panel. Direct these lengths straight up and cut. Work forward through this panel, releasing the horizontal sections and cutting to the traveling guide. Use pivotal partings through the crown area, cutting to the established length guide.

5. Direct front lengths back to create increased length. Repeat the technique on the other side of the head, then work through the center top to blend away the weight corner created. Note the curved finger position.

6. Use a cutting comb to taper the sides and back. Be careful not to cut into the previously cut length. Taper both sides, then continue tapering the entire nape area.

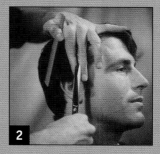
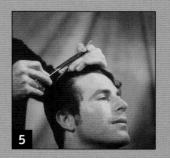
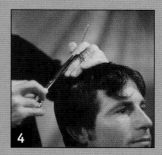
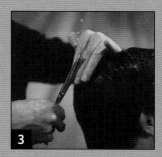
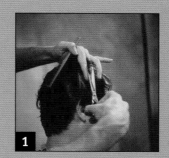
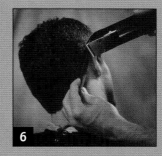

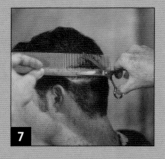

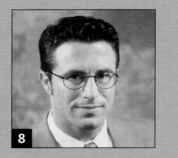

7. To create a smooth transition all around the hairline, refine and detail the cut, using a scissors-over-comb technique. Then style the hair into place.

8. The finished classic taper is a perfect business look.

CREATE

Apply this technique to different lengths, colors, and textures for almost endless possibilities.

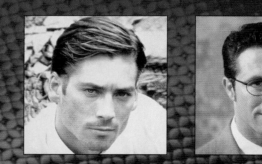